The Art Of Being Well

Tips To Improve Quality Of Health
(A guide book)

Compiled by
Syed Shaukat Islam Rizvi
Oakville ON Canada 2016

Index

A note ....

Very often, people believe that wellness is the same as health. This is not really the case. Health is a state of physical, mental, and social well-being. It involves more than just the absence of disease. A truly healthy person not only feels good physically but also has a realistic outlook on life and gets along well with other people. Good health enables people to enjoy life and have the opportunity to achieve the goals they have set for themselves. This is called wellness. There are many dimensions of wellness for living a healthy and balanced life. It is important to recognize that the dimensions are not independent of one another; they are interconnected. This means that factors affecting one dimension will often affect others. The following are some of the most important factors:

Emotional Wellness

An emotionally well person can freely express and manage their own feelings, thoughts, and behavior. They are aware of personal limitations, function well autonomously and understand the value of seeking support and assistance.

Intellectual Wellness

An intellectually well person incorporates what is learned in the classroom with what is experienced outside the classroom to enhance their potential for living a more fulfilling life.

Social Wellness

A socially well person lives in harmony with fellow human beings, seeks positive interdependent relationships with others, develops healthy behavior, and generally works for harmony in both personal and community environments.

Spiritual Wellness

A spiritually well person seeks meaning and purpose in human existence, questions everything, and appreciates and accepts the things that cannot be readily explained or understood. Being a Muslim, one should understand the purpose of our creation and follow the guidance given in the Quran and Sunnah. We have been given the wisdom and guidance for taking the right decisions in line with the Quran and Sunnah and we have the power and freedom to take the right decision for a better life in this world and in the hereafter.

Physical Wellness

A physically well person pursues an active lifestyle and understands the relationship between nutrition, activity, performance, and health.

Wellness is what comes after good health. Good health makes you feel normal; wellness makes you feel better than you were, both physically and mentally.

This document is compiled as a reference or guidebook to help achieve physical wellness – a good quality of health. The motivation to compile this document came from the recovery of my mysteriously long illness in 2005 when I was in a coma for 5 months, on the hospital bed for 8 months and practically paralyzed for year-and-a-half in USA. This illness made me appreciate the real value of good health and wellness. By the grace of Allah, family support, best-inclass medical treatment, prayers by hundreds of my friends, acquaintances, non-acquaintances and well-wishers and our faith in Allah. Alhamdullillah, I have regained all that I lost during illness. Since then I started reading, understanding and appreciating health-related articles. This compilation is a collection of some of those best articles from different sources. It is intended to be used as a reference book to improve the quality of health.

Shaukat Rizvi

April 2016

Rizvi's other works

Family Pentagon

Quranic Instructions for Daily Life

Hadith a Qudsi

This is How Thinking Negatively Will Affect Your Body

The 'Placebo Effect': you've probably heard about this mysterious term before. The body's ability to get better through nothing but sugar pills, saline injections or fake surgeries. And whilst according to clinical trials, most bodies do get better (18 to 80% of the time), there is a darker side to the seemingly mysterious placebo effect. In comparison, few people know about its evil twin, the 'Nocebo Effect', which holds the belief that negative emotions can potentially harm the body. But how exactly does it work?

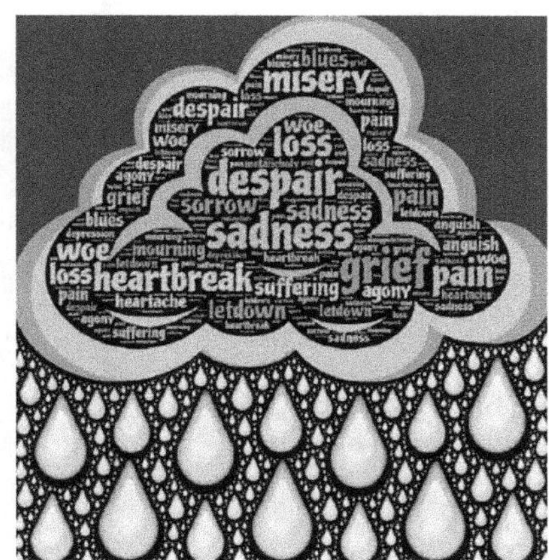

The mind-body connection

Your mind and mental state can have a profound effect on your physical body and your overall quality of life. And whilst it is possible to 'think yourself better', you may just as likely be able to 'think yourself sick'. Focusing your attention on illness has been scientifically proven to predispose the body to illness. When dealing with negative emotions such as anxiety, fear or an overall negative outlook on your health or life, these negative emotions trigger the amygdala in the limbic brain to send a red alert that activates the fight-or-flight stress response and when the nervous system is in 'fight-or-flight', the body's self repair mechanisms don't function properly, thus causing it to be predisposed to illness or pain.

How an emotional experience affected my body on a physical level

Two years ago I had a fall out with a dear friend. To me it felt like one of the most heartbreaking experiences I have ever had. Things hadn't ended well and for months I had experienced an array of negative emotions; anger, irritability, stress, overwhelming sadness - you name it. After 10 months of bombarding my body with these negative emotions, I began to experience a tightness in my upper and middle spine (find out more below) which after some time resulted in me having weekly panic attacks and a painful tightness within my chest - on occasion I had had two or three a week.

Whilst I did visit my GP to help deal with this issue, the panic attacks had actually stopped when I made peace with the situation. Now, this does not mean that I don't think about what happened, or that it doesn't saddens me from time to time, but rather that i've come to terms with the experience and all the negative emotions that came with it. I discovered that the more I addressed the unconscious thought pattern and emotions throughout my body, the more I found that the panic attacks subsided. So, what could the **possible** physical effects on your body be, which may have been a result of emotional pain and negative mental thought patterns?

Disclaimer: Whilst it is an intriguing and conceivable factor to look at physical pain on your body as a result of mental thought patterns, it is **ALWAYS IMPORTANT** to **SEEK PROFESSIONAL AND MEDICAL ADVICE FROM A DOCTOR.**

The mental-emotional-physical connection: Pain areas and probable causes

Neck	Refusing to see other sides of the question; stubbornness; inflexibility.
Shoulders	Represents our ability to carry our experiences in our life, joyously. We make life a burden by our attitude.
Spine	Represents the support of life.
Upper Spine	Represents lack of emotional support; feeling unloved; holding back love.
Middle Spine	Guilt; stuck in the past; a 'get off my back' attitude.
Lower Spine	Fear of money; lack of financial support
Elbows	Represents changing directions and accepting new experiences.
Wrists	Represents movement and ease.
Hips	Fear of going forward in major decisions; nothing to look forward to.
Knees	Stubborn pride and ego; inability to bend; fear; inflexibility; won't give in.
Ankles	Inflexibility and guilt; they represent the ability to receive pleasure.
Bunions	Lack of joy in meeting experiences in life.
Joint pain	Represents changes in direction in life and the ease of these movements.
Loss of balance	An inability to feel centered; scattered thinking.
Sciatica	Being hypocritical; fear of money and/or the future.
Slipped disk	Feel unsupported by life; feeling indecisive.
Stiffness	Rigid, stiff thinking.

Source: Information gathered from **Heal Your Body A-Z, Louise L. Hay**

Our emotional responses to our experiences may sometimes cloud our judgment and lead us on a downward- spiral, but rather than letting yourself feel overcome by your negative thoughts, take a moment to step back and observe the big picture. Bear in mind that each and every single experience, no matter how big or how small can help us see or learn something new, whilst also giving us the opportunity to clear an emotion within ourselves

Source: Flickr.com, Celestine Chua

Can Complaining Be Killing Us ?
(The Science Behind Your Everlasting Happiness Explained)

Did you know that if you complain about things frequently, you could actually be digging yourself an early grave? There is actual science to back this up, and what's even more astounding is the fact that you can actually shape your own reality with your thoughts. Read on to find out about the science of happiness:

1. **"Synapses that fire together wire together."**
   Synapses are structures that are present throughout the brain. They act as message relays for thoughts, speech and movement. When a thought pops into your head, a synapse fires a chemical across a tiny gap to another synapse. In other words, an electrical signal is built across a bridge in your brain. Every time the above occurs, your synapses grow closer together, meaning that the distance between them is reduced, allowing them to pass on the electrical signal quicker. The brain basically rewires its own circuitry, which means that your thoughts reshape your brain – literally.

2. **Shortest Path Wins the Race.**
   The synapses that bond most strongly together in your brain actually form your default personality – from your intelligence, to your skills and aptitude at different tasks in different situations. Furthermore, they determine what your most easily-accessible thoughts are, which has a great bearing on your conversational skills. The more a thought is repeated in your head, the closer together you bring the synapses that pass it on. The thought that wins the race inside your brain is the one that has the least distance to travel between synapses.

3. **Acceptance vs. Regret, Drift vs. Desire, Love vs. Fear.**
   Whenever the opportunity arises for us to think a reactive thought, you're generally faced with the following choices: Love versus Fear; Acceptance versus Regret; Drift versus Desire, or Optimism versus Pessimism. Taking the first example, you can choose to love everything in life while relinquishing your need for control. If you approach everything in your life from a perspective of love and do not try to control what you cannot, then you have nothing to fear. According to Buddhist philosophy, the universe itself is a place of suffering and chaos, thus our attempts to exert control over what goes on within it are nothing but futile. Practicing acceptance of the natural flow of life, giving thanks for each experience you have and every lesson you learn, will result in the synapses in your brain that represent love having a much higher chance of being triggered before those associated with sadness, regret, pessimism, fear, depression and so on. Repeatedly approaching situations from an optimistic and loving perspective will turn your default mental state into one of optimism and appreciation.With the above being said, you must note that this isn't a fool-proof practice. Sometimes the burden of emotion weighs too heavily on us, and being in a negative state of mind from time to time is just a part of life. However, just like any muscle in your body, you will see the results you want through regular, repeated exercise – you'll garner a new, innate strength, which will permeate your world with beauty.

4. **Mirror-Neurons**
   While it may be a revelation to you that you can actually shape your own reality with your thoughts, the thoughts of those around you can contribute greatly to it as well.
   When we observe someone experiencing a specific emotion, our brain tests out the emotion we perceive in order for us to try and understand what that person is going through. This is the basis of empathy, which although contains a whole world of good in itself, is also something that can have negative effects.
   Think of a mob mentality – when collective anger influences others to pick up their pitchforks against the common enemy, or listening to that annoying friend of yours who berates everyone and everything to gain some self-validation. In the latter instance, you find yourself reluctantly agreeing with them that yes, what they're complaining about really is unfair or just a load of baloney.
   The fact of the matter is that life is chaotic. If you continue to let the chaos that surrounds you influence you, then you're shaping your brain in such a way that your default, short-path personality will become bitter and jaded, rather than loving and optimistic.
   Spend time with people that elevate you – that are happy and full of love, rather than people that make you live in fear of being invalidated. This doesn't mean that you shouldn't help out friends who are going through a hard time, nor does it mean that you cannot critique the world's failings and injustices. After all, positive change usually requires critical thought.

5. **Stress is a killer.**

Negativity, regret, attachment to desire and pointless complaining about things that don't really matter will ultimately kill you. Although this point might seem drastic, all of these things ultimately lead to stress. When your brain is working away, firing angry synapses, your immune system gets weakened as a result and you'd be putting yourself at risk of a whole range of health problems.

The human stress hormone is called cortisol, and it's somewhat of a public enemy in the medical profession.

Elevated cortisol levels cause a decline in learning and memory, a decrease in immune function and bone density, an increase in weight gain, a rise in blood pressure and cholesterol levels, and a higher susceptibility to heart disease. These are just a few of the ailments that can be brought on by cortisol.

The Bottom Line

The universe is a chaotic place, and you happen to live in it. Each and every moment that you go through in your life has the potential to spawn other moments, ranging anywhere from soul-crushing grief, all the way to spirit-soaring bliss. The choice of where the majority of your future moments lie on that scale is really up to you.

Decide whether you're going to live in Love or Fear. It's obvious that life will always present you with moments of hardship, such as the passing of a loved one, the end of a romance or a failure in professional or academic life, but you don't have to live in regret of them when they do present themselves.

Don't feed these moments with negative attention – doing so will just make you cynical and jaded, blinding you to the fact that your very existence means you live in a cosmic playground, where you get to be the master of your own destiny through the choices you make.

When faced with a tough situation, be accepting of it. Say yes, this was horrible, but what have I learned from going through it? How is it going to make me a better person? How can I take strength from this so I can be closer to happiness in the next moment?

An example of the above is when a relationship ends. If there's something your ex used to do that drove you completely mad, you have the gift of knowing in the present not to waste any time on people who behave with you in the same way your ex used to.

Be mindful of the lessons you learn from your failures. Each day can be better than the one before it. Try something new every single day, live in love over fear, and strive to make your life better. The more you do these things, the more you will see how beautiful life really is, and ultimately, the happier you will be.

Ref: http://www.ba-bamail.com/

Behaviors That Harm Our Immune System

As you probably already know, the health of your immune system is actually YOUR health. The better it is off, the more resistant you are to invading viruses and infection. Many seem to think that the biggest influence on your immune system is vaccinations and diseases. This is only a small part of the story.

Your habits, those things you do daily, have a huge impact on your immune system and ultimately - on how protected you are from illness, especially as you get older. Here are 8 behaviors that damage your immune system and that you should avoid for your own good

1. **You don't chit-chat enough**

    It is becoming more and more clear that social interaction isn't just healthy for the mind but also for the body. The mere social behavior may contribute a lot to our well being. Research has shown that a low level of social interaction at home, work, and the community makes us more likely to become sick.

    When we lack social engagement, our brains get flooded with anxiety-generating chemicals, and we end up actually living shorter lives than our more sociable friends. One research that our of 270+ people between the ages of 18-55, those that had 6 or more regular social interactions were 4 times better at holding off cold viruses.

    How to solve: We all have hectic lives at times, but don't forget to cultivate and maintain your friendships, they may be just as important as your gym membership.

2. **You don't get enough sleep**

    There's always something to do, and this day and age - always something to watch. But staying up late and waking up early is associated by many health experts with a weak immune system that has a reduced amount of killer white blood cells to fight germs and viruses with. A study conducted by the University of Chicago found that men who sleep only 4 hours a night, for 1 week only, only produced half (!) the amount of antibodies designed to fight off flu, compared to those sleeping 7.5-8.5 hours per night.

    How to solve: Most adults require 7-9 hours of uninterrupted sleep per night, but if you're still tired half an hour after waking up - your quality of sleep is probably not so good. Try to get enough sleep and if you are tired - consult a sleep specialist, because sleep is crucial to your immune system and overall wellbeing.

3. **You're a downer**

    Serious research has unequivocally shown that people who tend to look at the glass as half empty and with a leak, have more stress in their lives and worse health. Those that are more optimistic have a higher T-cell count, a better immune response, and more powerful white cells. Now of course it could be that optimistic people take better care of themselves and their health, but it seems quite logical that a blacked look at life will cause your body to also get depressed, and with it your immune system.

    How to solve: It's not that easy to just clap your hands and poof! you're an optimist. It takes a real commitment to change your speech and thought patterns, simply by asking yourselves: "what other way can I look at this? Is there a less terrible way to judge this?" Try it, a little at a time. Try to really understand why something, or someone, might be better than you thought. Change will come with time, and with it - a boost to your immune system.

4. **You fight with your spouse in the wrong way**

    A very interesting research by UCLA found that couples that discuss their problems openly receive the same boost to their immune system and killer cell count as they would get from mild exercise. On the flip side, couples that fight by sarcasm, insults and passive-aggressive behavior have less T cells, higher levels of stress hormones (logically) and may take up to 40% loner to recover from injuries than their more open and positive counterparts. **How to solve:** Habits and relationship dynamics are also hard things to change, and many couples rely on friendly banter. That's fine, it is when that banter becomes a bit TOO sharp that you start suffering, and it's never good for the relationship either. If you have a real problem, discussing it bravely and openly with your spouse is not just healthy for your relationship, but apparently also for your own body.

5. **No break from the rat race of stress**

    Everyone deals with stress on occasion, but what happens when we are under stress day after day, with hardly any letup? What happens is that your immune system starts experiencing a decline in its ability to fight infection, virus and germ. Periods of stress that do not let up quickly will cause your killer cell count to drop and turn your immune system more sluggish. It is a known fact that widows and widowers are a lot more likely to get sick in the year following the death of their spouse than those who have not gone through this major loss and stress-inducing event.

How to solve: To each their own. We all have things that relieve our stress, whether it's a scented bath, going to the gym, getting off work for a few days or anything in between. Remember those things that relax you and go do them on a regular basis. That's right, make room in your busy calender for 'relaxation' - that is if you want to live a healthier life.

6. You borrow stuff from other people

Take our advice: If you need to use a pen, bring your own. If you need a calculator, bring your own. If you need a laptop... well, you get the point. Cold and flu germs are passed, more often than not, by hand to hand contact. You never know where an object has been and who has touched it. We're not saying run away when someone offers you a pen, but we would suggest not making a habit of borrowing other people's stuff - you never know when you might pick something up and pass it along to your family.

How to solve: Make a list of the most common items you will need to use during the day. Carry a bag or have some deep pockets for some basic stuff like a pen. Don't borrow stuff that you can bring from home.

7. Leave those antibiotics alone

Antibiotics were invented to fight serious infections and germs. Taking antibiotics every time you have a slight illness or a few symptoms will cause your body to develop a more serious resistance to antibiotics, and so you will become vulnerable to the more serious cases of infection. Research has found that patients tending to take a lot of antibiotics have a more suppressed immune system, which means you will get more sick in the future, so you are just postponing this light sickness for a more serious illness down the line.

How to solve: Only take antibiotics when you have a bacterial infection, take as much as ordered, but do not use them to prevent illness unless instructed to specifically by your doctor. Don't save antibiotics you didn't use for the future, use as much as told and throw away the rest.

8. Why so serious?

This may be no laughing matter, but your immune system loves a good chuckle. Research has shown that emotions accompanying real laughter cause a decrease in the level of stress hormones in the body as well as certain immune cells. In a recent research conducted at the Loma Lina University of Medicine, adults watching a funny video for as little as an hour showed significant increases in their immune system activity.

How to solve: Well, we think this one explains itself! **Laughmore**, people! Enjoy your favorite comedies, meet with your funniest friends, read silly comics and memes and just open yourself to funny experiences!

Ref: http://www.ba-bamail.com/

21 Rules For a Good Old Age

Some of us have reached our golden years, and some of us have not. But these suggestions should be read by everyone. They have been collected from many a senior, each with his or her own piece of advice. Some you may know, some may surprise you, and some will remind you of what's important. So read well, share with your loved ones, and have a great day and a great life!

1. It's time to use the money you saved up. Use it and enjoy it. Don't just keep it for those who may have no notion of the sacrifices you made to get it. Remember there is nothing more dangerous than a son or daughter-in-law with big ideas for your hard earned capital. Warning: This is also a bad time for an investment, even if it seems wonderful or fool-proof. They only bring problems and worries and this is a time for you to enjoy some peace and quiet.

2. Stop worrying about the financial situation of your children and grandchildren, and don't feel bad spending your money on yourself. You've taken care of them for many years, and you've taught them what you could. You gave them an education, food, shelter and support. The responsibility is now theirs to earn their own money.

3. Keep a healthy life, without great physical effort. Do moderate exercise (like walking every day), eat well and get your sleep. It's easy to become sick, and it gets harder to remain healthy. That is why you need to keep yourself in good shape and be aware of your medical and physical needs. Keep in touch with your doctor, get tested even when you're feeling well. Stay informed.

4. Always buy the best, most beautiful items for your significant other. The key goal is to enjoy your money with your partner. One day one of you will miss the other, and the money will not provide any comfort then, enjoy it together.

5. Don't stress over the little things. You've already overcome so much in your life. You have good memories and bad ones, but the important thing is the present. Don't let the past drag you down and don't let the future frighten you. Feel good in the now. Small issues will soon be forgotten.

6. Regardless of age, always keep love alive. Love your partner, love life, love your family, love your neighbor and remember: "A man is not old as long as he has intelligence and affection."

7. Be proud, both inside and out. Don't stop going to your hair salon or barber, do your nails, go to the dermatologist and the dentist, keep your perfumes and creams well stocked. When you are well-maintained on the outside, it seeps in, making you feel proud and strong.

8. Don't lose sight of fashion trends for your age, but keep your own sense of style. There's nothing worse than an older person trying to wear the current fashion among youngsters. You've developed your own sense of what looks good on you - keep it and be proud of it. It's part of who you are.

9. ALWAYS stay up-to-date. Read newspapers, watch the news. Go online and read what people are saying. Make sure you have an active email account and try to sign up to a couple of social networks. You'll be surprised which old friends you may meet. Keeping in touch with what is going on and with the people you know, is important at any age.

10. Respect the younger generation and their opinions. They may not have the same ideals as you, but they are the future, and will take the world in their direction. Give advice, not criticism, and try to remind them of yesterday's wisdom that still applies today.

11. Never use the phrase: "In my time". Your time is now. As long as you're alive, you are a part of this time. Have fun and enjoy life.

12. Some people embrace their golden years, while others become bitter and surly. Life is too short to waste your days on the latter. Spend your time with positive, cheerful people, it'll rub off on you and your days will seem that much better. Spending your time with bitter people will make you older and harder to be around.

13. Do not surrender to the temptation of living with your children or grandchildren (if you have a financial choice, that is). Sure, being surrounded by family sounds great, but we all need our privacy. They need theirs and you need yours. If you've lost your partner (our deepest condolences), then find a person to move in with you and help out. Even then, do so only if you feel you really need the help or do not want to live alone.

14. Don't abandon your hobbies. If you don't have any, make new ones. You can travel, hike, cook, read, dance. You can adopt a cat or a dog, grow a garden, play cards, checkers, chess, dominoes, golf. You can paint, volunteer at an NGO or just collect certain items. Find something you like and spend some real time having fun with it.

15. Even if you don't feel like it, try to accept invitations. Baptisms, graduations, birthdays, weddings, conferences. Try to go. Get out of the house, meet people you haven't seen in a while, experience something new (or something old). But don't get upset when you're not invited. Some events are limited by resources, and not everyone can be hosted. The important thing is to leave the house from time to time. Go to museums, go walk through a field. Get out there.

16. Be a conversationalist. Talk less and listen more. Some people go on and on about the past, not caring if their listeners are really interested. That's a great way of reducing their desire to speak with you. Listen first and answer questions, but don't go off into long stories unless asked to. Speak in courteous tones and try not to complain or criticize too much unless you really need to. Try to accept situations as they are. Everyone is going through the same things, and people have a low tolerance for hearing complaints. Al
ways find some good things to say as well.

17. Pain and discomfort go hand in hand with getting older. Try not to dwell on them but accept them as a part of the cycle of life we're all going through. Try to minimize them in your mind. They are not who you are, they are something that life has added to you. If they become your entire focus, you lose sight of the person you used to be.

18. If you've been offended by someone - forgive them. If you've offended someone - apologize. Don't drag around resentment with you. It only serves to make you sad and bitter. It doesn't matter who was right. Someone once said: "Holding a grudge is like taking poison and expecting the other person to die." Don't take that poison. Forgive, forget and move on with your life.

19. If you have a strong belief, savor it. But don't waste your time trying to convince others. They will make their own choices no matter what you tell them, and it will only bring you frustration. Live your faith and set an example. Live true to your beliefs and let that memory sway them.

20. Laugh. Laugh A LOT. Laugh at everything. Remember, you are one of the lucky ones. You've managed to have a life, a long one. Many never get to this age, never get to experience a full life. But you did. So what's not to laugh about? Find the humor in your situation.

21. Take no notice of what others say about you and even less notice of what they might be thinking. They'll do it anyway, and you should have pride in yourself and what you've achieved. Let them talk and don't worry. They have no idea about your history, your memories and the life you've lived so far. There's still much to be written, so get busy writing and don't waste time thinking about what others might think. Now is the time to be at rest, at peace and as happy as you can be!

AND REMEMBER: "Life is too short to drink bad wine."

Ref: http://www.ba-bamail.com/

Popular False Myths in Health

If you're on the look-out for what to eat and what to avoid, you've probably been given some advice from colleagues, friends and family members that sounds reliable. If you're taking it super seriously, you might have even looked up diet tips on blogs or online forums. We've all been lent some genius expertise, which by all means, sound pretty obvious and credible. Well…after you read the following facts (backed up by scientific research) you'll realize just how gullible you might have been to believe these common food myths.

1. **"Eating fatty food makes you fat."**
This is a wide-spread misconception, which leads dieting individuals to substitute their seemingly fatty intake with portions of greens. In reality, consuming fatty food does not mean you will become fat, or that the fat will be trapped in your body. Balance is the key. Even though some fats are considered 'worse' than others, excess intake of any kind of food in general may lead to weight gain, including carbohydrates and protein. Here's what Dr. Carly Stewart (medical expert at Money Crashers) states about the matter: "Eating fatty foods does not make you fat. Fat in moderation is a necessary part of any healthy and balanced diet. Putting on more weight in the form of fat is a result of energy imbalance. You will gain weight if you take in more calories than you burn. Fat is a concentrated source of calories, but it is not necessary to eliminate fat from your diet completely."
Bottom line: **Fat won't make you fat, unless you eat too much of it.** So go ahead and fill your plate with varied foods, and put your mind at rest. All you need to do is maintain a healthy balance.
Learn more about fat in our article: Did you know: What is fat?

2. **"Eating carbs makes you fat."**
Ok, we've debunked the 'fat makes you fat' myth. But what about carbohydrates? Are these tempting donuts, for instance, to blame for our flabby stomachs? t of all, carbohydrates aren't only sugar, they also come in forms of starch and fiber. This means that when peo they'll eliminate carbs from their diet, they're also including fruits, vegetables, milk, nuts, grains, seeds and mes, all of which are super vital for our body. So, what's the right thing to do? This is what Dr. Stewart mmends:
" is a good idea to limit the number of carbs you eat in the form of sugar because sugar is low in nutritional val high in calories. However, if you eliminate carbs completely, you will miss out on healthy food such as whole n breads and wheat pastas. You will only gain weight if you consume more calories than you burn."
Bottom line: **Eliminating carbs entirely from your diet is wrong.** They will only make you fat if you have a poor diet or lack of exercise. Some carbs are less healthy than others, such as sugary and processed foods, but this does not mean you should remove them from your diet. Again, keeping a reasonable balance is a must, alongside regular exercise.
Learn more about carbs in our article: How Carbs, Not Fat, are Making You Fatter

3. **"Gluten-free food is healthier."**
Being gluten-intolerant means you may need to cut down on your intake of quite a number of produce, including bread, pasta, cereal, beer, pastries, etc. Of course, there are gluten-free alternatives to these, which lately have not only been used by people who suffer from this intolerance , but also by people who believe this myth. Just as some people find they feel better when eating gluten-free products, these products are not always a healthy option since they are often made with refined starches. Here's what Dr. Stewart suggests:
" Gluten-free foods are only healthier for you if you are allergic to gluten. If you aren't, eating a gluten-free diet tricts the amount of fiber, vitamins, and minerals you are able to consume. A variety of foods that are high in ole grains (such as foods containing wheat, rye, or barley) also contain gluten, and these foods are an essential t of a healthy diet. Most people have no trouble digesting gluten. "
Bottom line: **Only unless you are sensitive or allergic to gluten, there's absolutely nothing wrong in consuming it.** Don't miss out on nutrients you are able to tolerate just because you were carried away with one of the gluten myths. Go ahead and enjoy your beer, without needing to worry - and as always, don't forget: balance.
Learn more about gluten in our article: What the Heck is Gluten?

4. **"Everyone needs to defecate daily."**
You might have grown concerned when hearing people say that they're able to defecate twice a day, and asked yourself - how is that even possible? If you're not as efficient as them, does that mean you have something wrong? Well, these people have been honest enough with you and yes, many might need more frequent use of the toilet than others. But this doesn't mean there's something wrong with your body.
According to Dr. Stewart, everyone has different schedules:
❝ No single bowel movement schedule is right for everyone. However, staying hydrated, eating foods high in er, and being active will help ensure that your schedule is regular and you do not become backed up. ❞
Bottom line: **As long as your stool is healthy, you needn't worry about how frequent you poop.** This frequency might even depend on your food and water intake. Unless you're feeling any discomfort or are seriously constipated, you can put your mind at rest.
Learn more about digestion in our article: 14 Tips to Naturally Improve Your Digestive System

5. **"The microwave kills nutrients in food."**
Most of us might be familiar with this myth, and with the microwave being so widely-used nowadays, it has also become quite a worry to families, especially because they've been told microwaves can kill nutrients in food. People might not have been completely wrong on this, but there's certainly nothing to worry about. Dr. Spencer Nadolsky (medical editor at Examine.com) elaborates on this:
❝ Microwaving can kill some nutrients (sulforaphane from broccoli, for example) but this does not extend to all trients. Unfortunately, we need to look at this stuff on a case by case basis to see which foods you should crowave and which you cannot since there is no rhyme or reason to which compounds are damaged or ctivated. In general, microwaving is not a serious concern. ❞
Bottom line: **There's no major reason to abandon your microwave.** You might be more concerned about your microwave not heating meals evenly or not keeping your food in the desired texture, rather than it killing nutrients. After all, heating up broccoli in any way will cause it to lose its sulforaphane.

6. **"Spot training helps you burn fat in desired areas."**
Everyone has stubborn areas in their body that gain weight more easily than others, such as the stomach, legs or arms. People who have always wanted to target those areas in weight loss have tried 'spot training', but the fact that it's not effective might not be well received by these individuals. The reality is explained by Dr. Stewart:
❝ Doing sit-ups (or another type of spot training) will strengthen the abdominal muscles, but will not burn fat specific to that area. Fat is burned or lost throughout the body on a more even basis, and is accomplished through aerobic or cardiovascular exercise. The pattern of fat gain or loss has more to do with each person's unique body than it does with the type of aerobic exercise performed. ❞
Bottom line: **Spot training won't help you eliminate fat from specific areas.** However, this should in no way stop you from doing it. Muscle building makes you fit and it is still beneficial to burn fat in any part of your body.

7. **"The scale is a good way to see your fat loss progress."**
So you've lost a pound or 2, and you're feeling satisfied. Your desired results are finally showing numeric proof on the scale - you're definitely burning enough fat! Wait - are you sure it's fat you're losing? The truth is, our body is made of much more than just fat. We all know it consists of a large quantity of water for starters, together with other materials, which can also be lost after exercise. Dr. Stewart explains further:
❝ The scale treats both fat and muscle the same way – a pound of fat is the same as a pound of muscle. If you're engthening your muscles during your exercise regimen, you might actually see a small amount of weight gain her than weight loss, which is not a bad thing. A better way to track the progress of diet and exercise is to onitor how you feel and how you look. Your local fitness center mayalso be able to help with measuring your rcent body fat. ❞
Bottom line: **Using the scale is not the best way to track the progress of your diet.** It may mislead you in both positive and negative ways - you may be interpreting muscle gain as fat gain, or water loss as fat loss. But either way, you will probably realize when you'd been burning your fat by the way you see yourself and feel.

Ref: H/T: Lifehacker.com

Control Your Weight with these 20 Tips

In my younger years, I was obsessed with eating low-fat food and less carbohydrates. But over time, I've come to learn that there is more to weight loss than a low-fat diet. True, to lose weight you need to watch what you eat, but I have found that in adopting certain lifestyle changes and including more wholesome food into my diet, I have managed to maintain my weight. These 20 tips, backed by science, have worked exceptionally well for me.

1. **Control your portions by eating from small plates**

   Research has shown that people eat less when served food on a small plate instead of a large one. Scientists believe that eating from a plate which looks full will trick the mind into believing that you are eating more. To control your portion further, scientists believe that eating from blue plates may cause you to eat less than plates of other colors - the reason why this works is unclear.

Use this Calorie Control Guide to help you decipher how much you should eat.

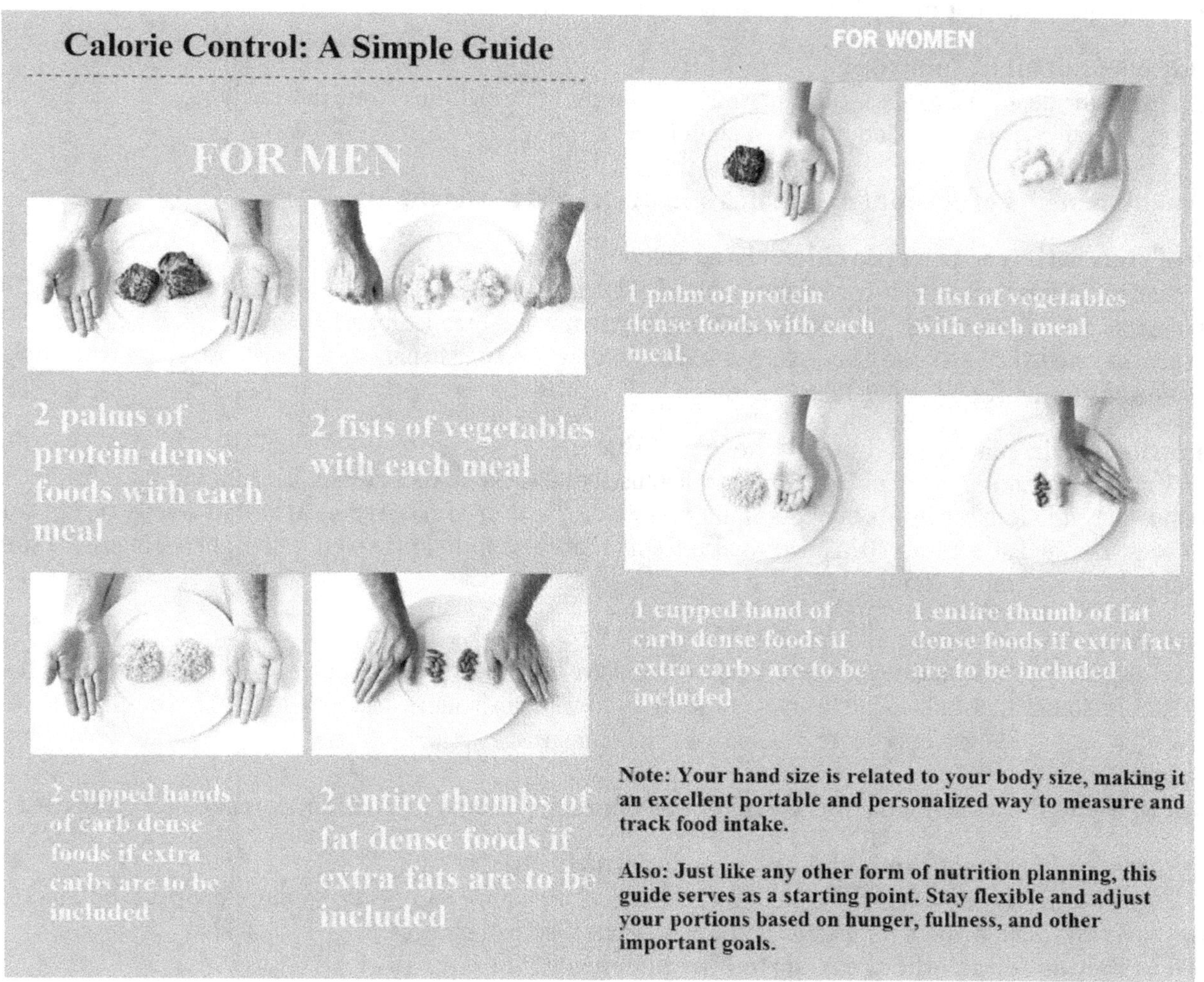

2. **Make sure you're getting enough sleep**

   Being sleep-deprived can lower levels of leptin (an appetite-suppressing hormone) while increasing ghrelin (a hunger-stimulating hormone). Consequently, those who are sleep-deprived tend to be hungrier and crave junk foods like carbs, candy and salty foods. Furthermore, studies have shown that women who go to bed and wake up at the same time every day have lower levels of body fat.

3. **Reduce your stress and anxiety to keep your hormones balanced**

   When we feel stressed, our bodies release a hormone called cortisol. If elevated for too long, it leads to an increase in the amount of visceral fat around the tummy. Still, cortisol isn't the only hormone that messes with your weight. The thyroid and adrenals play a part too. If our hormones are out of sync, we can find it more difficult to lose weight. **If you've been feeling a little stressed lately, try these 8 pressure point techniques. (see it on later pages)**

4. **Trick your way into feeling full by smelling your food**
Several studies have shown that smelling your food may be enough to trick your brain into feeling full. Satiating smells include extra virgin olive oil, garlic, apples, bananas, fennel and grapefruit.

5. **Avoid buying fruits and vegetables that contain pesticides**
A Canadian study conducted on mice found that chemicals in pesticides slow down metabolic function, increasing the risk of obesity and diabetes. A better alternative would be to buy organic food.

6. **Allow yourself a cheat day each week**
According to research conducted, a cheat meal once a week can rev up the metabolism by reviving levels of leptin, balancing thyroid hormones and reducing cravings. As much as possible, try to keep it healthy and choose high carb over high-fat meals for a high leptin effect.

7. **Don't eat when you are distracted**
A paper published in the American Journal of Clinical Nutrition reports that multitasking while eating (whether you are watching television, driving or working) or eating in a hurry may cause you to eat more.

8. **Include coconut oil in your diet**
Aside from being delicious, coconut oil contributes a great deal to weight loss. You can add it to your baked goods, use it to fry, use it as a coffee creamer, or add it to your smoothies.

    The health benefits of coconut oil are not only restricted to weight loss.

9. **Control your satiety with apple cider vinegar**
Apple cider vinegar is well known for balancing blood sugar levels and satiety. In one study, participants were given varying levels of apple cider vinegar with carbohydrates in the form of white bread. Blood test shows that the higher the levels of apple cider ingested, the lower the blood glucose and insulin levels of participants. Furthermore, those who consumed the most vinegar reported feeling fuller than the others.

10. **Use mushroom in place of red meat where possible**
Mushrooms are a great replacement for red meat when used in dishes like cottage pies, lasagnas and tacos. In one study, it was found that individuals who ate one cup of mushrooms each day instead of red meat lost an average of 7 pounds, had a smaller waist size, and also a lower BMI. It was also found that these individuals were better able to maintain their weight loss than individuals who ate meat.

11. **Include avocados into your daily diet**
Avocados are rich in monounsaturated fatty acids, which have been shown to be a powerful reducer of belly fat. Studies conducted also found that individuals who ate fresh avocado with their lunch had 40% less desire to snack over the course of three hours and a 28% less desire over a period of five hours after a meal.

    Besides its weight loss benefits, there are plenty of other reasons to include avocados in your diet.

12. **Eating eggs for breakfast can help keep your weight down**
Research has found that eating eggs for breakfast can limit calorie intake for the day by more than 400 calories. Ideally, opt for free-range eggs as they have a far greater nutritional value than battery eggs.
(See Food section for 10 other reasons to introduce eggs into your diet.)

13. **Include spices in your diet to keep your weight down**
Herbs and spices are packed with antioxidants and are beneficial to the body in many ways. Some of them can also promote weight loss. These include:

    - **Garlic:** Studies show that rats fed a diet high in fat, alongside a garlic supplement, were found to have reduced weight and fat levels. It was also found that their blood and liver were safeguarded from the effects of not eating well.
    - **Cinnamon:** Studies have found cinnamon to be a powerful appetite suppressant. In fact, studies show that adding a small amount to carbohydrates may keep you full for longer.
    - **Cayenne Pepper:** A substance in cayenne called capsaicin, has been found to suppress hunger and increase satiety. Cayenne pepper has also been found to have thermo-genetic properties which can lead to increased metabolism.

- **Mint**: Some studies have found that just smelling mint can lead to eating significantly fewer calories.
- **Ginger**: In one study, individuals who drank 2 grams of ginger powder in hot water were less hungry three hours later than participants who didn't drink it.

14. Drink more spinach smoothies

According to studies conducted on spinach smoothies, drinking a spinach shake in the morning can reduce the effects of feeling hungry throughout the day, promoting weight loss.
Stocking up on spinach smoothies will do more for your body than help you lose weight.

15. Opt for dark chocolate

Just because you are trying to lose weight, doesn't mean that you don't deserve a treat every once in a while. But, if you feel the urge to indulge, go for some dark chocolate. One study found that individuals who ate dark chocolate instead of white experienced lower blood sugar levels - the key to losing and maintaining weight.
(See in food section 10 more reasons to take a bite out of dark chocolate.)

16. Opt for wholegrain carbohydrates as opposed to white

Stick to whole grain (brown) versions of bread, pasta and rice to help maintain your weight. A study conducted in 2008 found that participants who ate whole grain produce enjoyed greater reductions in weight, body mass and body fat, when compared to those who ate refined (white) carbohydrates. Whole grain foods are rich in fiber - an essential nutrient when trying to lose weight.

17. Blueberries are good for you

Rich in antioxidants, blueberries are packed with goodness. A study conducted in 2011 found that mice who consumed a handful of blueberries had a 73% decrease in fat lipids. Other research also found that meals enriched in blueberries saw greater levels of abdominal fat loss in rats.

18. Eat a bowl of oatmeal every morning

Starting your day off with a bowl of oatmeal will help regulate your blood sugar levels throughout the day, boosting your metabolism after a night's rest. Be sure to stay away from instant oatmeal - one serving can contain up to 17g of sugar.

19. If your cravings are getting the best of you, snack on pears and apples

Snack on fruits between meals. Pears and apples, in particular, contain a type of soluble fiber which reduces the amount of sugar and calories absorbed by the bloodstream after a meal, which in turn prevents fat storage and keeps you feeling full.
Snacking on apples between meals will also help fend off a number of diseases.

20. Coffee has a number of surprising benefits, including weight loss

Coffee is predominantly known to boost energy and brain function. It has also been found to lower the risk of diabetes and dementia. Studies have also discovered that coffee can increase your metabolism by up to 20% after drinking.

Ref: http://www.ba-bamai

11 Things We Do that Age Us

Aging gracefully comes easily to some, and less easily to others. Sometimes it's just to do with having good genes, but often it is the decisions we make during our lifetime that determine how fast we'll age. You may not realize it, but most people make mistakes every single day that make them age faster than they should, harming their skin and quickening the appearance of old age.

1. **You try to do too many things at once (Multitasking).**
   If your to-do list is longer than your arm and you are dealing with the stress of juggling many projects or tasks at once, you're doing yourself a disservice, says Raymond Casciari, Chief Medical Officer at St. Joseph Hospital. Several studies have shown that day-to-day stress triggers the release of free radicals in the body, which damage cells and quicken the aging process. The doctor suggests focusing on one task at a time.

2. **You rarely pass on dessert.**
   Other than being an obviously unhealthy habit, having a sweet tooth may be adding years to your face, as sugar molecules attach themselves to protein fibers in our cells, a process known as glycation. This can lead to an ashen look, dark circles around the eyes, a loss of facial contours, wrinkles, puffiness and bigger pores. So if you want to hold on to that youthful glow, don't overdo the sugar.

3. **You get less than 5-6 hours of sleep a night.**
   Not getting enough sleep doesn't only give you black bags under your eyes, but has been linked, through several studies, to a shorter life span. According to Dr. Casciari, the founder of a sleep lab at St. Joseph Hospital, getting about seven hours of sleep is optimal. So if you're nodding off, low on energy or finding it hard to focus, you're probably not sleeping enough, and it may age you faster than you'd like.

4. **You spend most of your day sitting.**
   Sitting and leading a sedentary lifestyle are some of the worst contributors to aging people in the modern world. Most people do very little physical activity, and the result is an increased risk of kidney disease, cardiovascular disease, cancer and of course obesity. Studies show that people who exercised 150 minutes a week or more lived 10-13 years longer on average.

5. **You don't use any eye creams.**
   The skin around your eyes is thinner than the rest of your face, and that is why it usually starts showing signs of aging sooner. Keeping the eye area moisturized can take years off your face. The best creams contain Retin-A, which is a form of vitamin A. But you can also add antioxidants, hyaluronic acid and vitamin C.

6. **You only use sunscreen when on vacation.**
   If you only use sunscreen at the beach, note that you may actually be doing more harm to your skin while running errands and driving. Skin damage accumulates, and the sun's rays are the primary reason for aging skin. Dr Taylor, associate professor of dermatology, recommends that you use an SPF between 30-50 for daily protection.

7. **You wear too much makeup.**
   This is not a judgment, just a fact. Many make-up products are oil-based, and can clog your pores and cause outbreaks. Overusing skin products with fragrances, alcohol agents and chemicals that irritate may cause premature lines and wrinkles.

8. **You sleep with your face against the pillow.**
   Sleeping on your stomach or side with your face mashed into the pillow may create wrinkles and make you age faster. Our facial skin gets less flexible with time, and so as we lie on the pillow night after night, our skin may not spring back and smooth the lines you had, and so the pillow can leave permanent marks on our face. So sleep on your back or invest in a satin pillowcase that'll keep your skin smooth.

9. **You keep your house very warm.**
   When you turn up the thermostat or light a fireplace because it's cold, it's tempting to make it hot and toasty inside. But the problem is that the thermostat, and also the fireplace, suck moisture out of the air in the house, which leads to dry skin. If this goes on, as indeed in cold climates it may, it will lead to damaged skin with aging effects. Invest in a humidifier, and set it to 40-60% humidity. This will free your skin from the itching, scratching and even flaking that comes with dry air. Another way to go is placing a wet towel over a radiator or a bowl of cold water in the room.

10. **You purse your lips**

Drinking your beverages through a straw can help you avoid staining your teeth, but just like squinting can give you wrinkles around the eyes, so can pursing your lips give you wrinkles around the mouth. By the way, this also often happens when you smoke a cigarette.

11. **You've stopped eating fat altogether.**

Some amounts of fat are required to maintain a youthful appearance and feeling, according to Franci Cohen, nutritionist and exercise physiologist from Brooklyn, NY. Heart healthy Omega 3 fatty acids, which you can find in oily fish such as mackerel and salmon, as well as nuts like walnuts and flax seeds, will keep your skin plump and supple. This will prevent wrinkles while also boosting the health of both your brain and heart. **Here are 11 mistakes we all make that age us**

Ref: http://www.ba-bamail.com/

How to Trick Your Body into Feeling Better

There are quite a few irritating and annoying sensations your body experiences during the day, the kind that most of us would love to know how to get rid of. For instance, how does one deal with an itchy throat? How do you make a burn go away? And generally, how can you get rid of various pains? This list will teach you how to treat all of these issues with relative ease.

1. **Itchy Throat? Scratch Your Ear**
   An itchy throat is a nuisance, and one that is difficult to get rid of unless you know this trick. When the inside of your throat feels itchy, it's virtually impossible to scratch, and in many cases, a loud cough is not socially acceptable. Luckily, the throat and ears are part of the same system, and according to Dr. Schaffer, Head Otolaryngologist in *Advocare*, NJ, when you stimulate the nerves in the ear, you create a reflexive reaction in the throat, causing it to contract, relieving the itch.

2. **The Right Ear Processes Speech More Effectively**
   Researchers from UCLA Medical School found that the right ear can process the faster rhythm of speech better than the left one. The left ear, on the other hand, is much more efficient at processing music. If you want to hear someone speaking in a crowd, try turning your right ear towards them. If you're attempting to listen to a song or melody, use your left ear.

3. **Mind Over Bladder**
   According to Dr. Larry Lipshultz, Head of Urology in the Baylor College of Medicine, if a man feels the need to urinate but doesn't have the opportunity – he can think about sex. By keeping your mind on sexual thoughts, you distract your body from the need to urinate, since the two cannot co-exist. It is important to remember that holding your bodily functions for too long is unhealthy and even dangerous, so be sure to relieve yourself as soon as possible.

4. **Coughing is a Painkiller**
   Pain is the body's way of warning us about damage to the body, but sometimes this warning is more of a distraction than helpful. Surprisingly, it's very easy to overcome. Researchers from Germany discovered that when patients were asked to cough while being injected, they felt no pain. The reason is that once you cough, your body increases the pressure in your chest and spine. This pressure blocks pain signals from moving up the spine, effectively working as a painkiller.

5. **Use Your Tongue to Ease Congestion**
   You can find plenty of decongestants at your local pharmacy, but there's an easy, natural alternative. What you need to do is alternate between using your tongue to push up against the roof of your mouth and applying pressure between your eyebrows using your finger. This action "shakes" the nasal bone, releasing the congestion within 20 seconds.

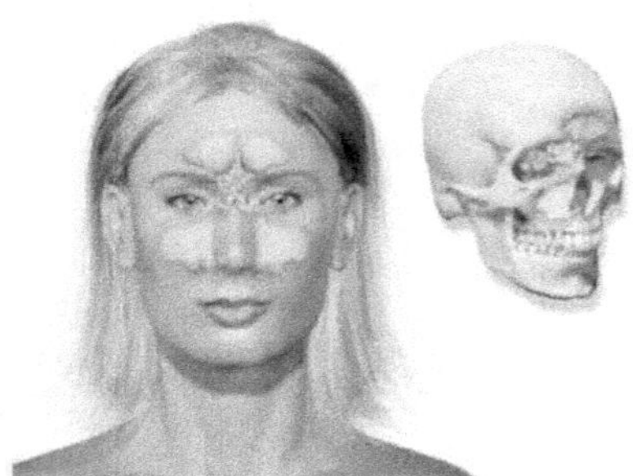

6. **Sleep on Your Left Side to Prevent Acid Reflux**
   According to Dr. Anthony Strippoli, a Gastroenterologist from Florida several studies have shown that by sleeping on your side you reduce the likeliness of suffering from heartburn. The esophagus and stomach are connected at a particular angle. If you lie on your right side, your stomach is positioned higher than your esophagus, making it easier for stomach acids to travel between them, causing heartburn. If you lie down on your left side, however, the stomach now rests below the esophagus, which will prevent stomach acids from escaping.

7. **Rub Ice on Your Hand to Relieve a Toothache**
   A Canadian study discovered an interesting phenomenon: When you rub ice on the back of your hand, between the area that connects the thumb and the forefinger, you can reduce the intensity of toothaches by up to 50%. The nerves in that part of the hand stimulate a part of the brain that blocks pain signals coming from the face and hands.

8. **Make Burn Blisters Vanish**
We're taught to put ice on burns to reduce their intensity, but the truth is that lukewarm temperatures work better. If you've gotten burned, clean the affected area and apply light pressure to the spot with the pads of your fingers, and run it under lukewarm water. While ice will numb the pain, returning the area to the normal temperature will prevent swelling and blistering.

9. **Stop "The Spins" When You're Drunk/Hungover**
The Cupula helps us maintain our balance. It is located in our ear, suspended in a liquid and has the same density as blood. When you drink too much alcohol, it dilutes the blood in the cupula, making it lighter than the liquid it is in, which in turn makes it float. This unnatural behavior confuses the brain and causes a loss of balance. To stop this from happening, you need to provide the brain with a "second opinion" – place both hands on a stable, horizontal surface. This will give your brain another source of stability to rely on, thanks to the sensitive nerves in your hands.

10. **Prevent "Stitches" When You Run**
Most people have experienced the feeling of "stitches" while running - a sharp, intense pain in your side - which makes it hard to breath. This often occurs because we exhale when our right foot hits the ground, putting pressure on the liver. The pressure on the liver causes it to "pull" on the diaphragm, making it very difficult to breath. To prevent this from happening, make sure you exhale when your left foot hits the ground.

11. **Safely Stop a Nosebleed**
If you get a nosebleed, most people would tell you to tilt your head back and apply pressure to your nose. While this method seems logical, it is actually quite dangerous, especially for children. When we tilt our head back, the blood flows down and may enter the respiratory system, which can cause suffocation and even death. A less-known, but far safer method, is to apply pressure with your thumb and forefinger on both sides of your nose, where the bone ends. Alternatively, you can place a piece of cotton wool on the inside of your upper lip, right at the center of the gums.

12. **Slow Your Pulse Through Breathing**
Whenever you get over-excited, and you feel like your heart is about to burst out of your chest, you can slow it down with a simple breathing technique. The nerve in charge of your heart rate is the Vagus Nerve, which can be controlled by rhythmic breathing. All you need to do is place the tips of your thumbs on your lips, and breathe through them (to slow down your breathing).

13. **Quickly Stop a "Brain Freeze."**
If you enjoy a frozen treat from time to time, you've probably experienced the irritating pain of "brain freeze". When you first eat something frozen, you shock the nerves in your mouth, which confuses your brain into thinking it's freezing. To compensate, your body heats up instantly, causing intense pain. To relieve this sensation, push your tongue against the roof of your mouth, making sure to cover as much space as possible. The more pressure you apply, the faster the pain will dissipate.

14. **Improve Your Eyesight**
In many cases, nearsightedness is the result of strain on the eye muscles, which occurs due to the discrepancy between our natural field of vision and the demands of modern life. In other words, staring at screens too closely can lead to eye muscles stiffening, making it harder to see objects that are further away.
Since we can't directly control our eye muscles, we can relax them by using a roundabout technique. By relaxing other muscle groups in your body, you can trigger a relaxation of the eye muscles. Close your eyes, take a deep breath and hold it in for a few seconds. When you exhale, loosen the muscles in your body. Another way to do this is by flexing and releasing your arm muscles, or your buttocks.

15. **Last Longer Under Water**
When we dive, it's not the lack of oxygen that makes us desperate for air. Instead, it's the accumulation of CO_2 in our blood. To extend the time it takes the CO_2 to accumulate in your blood, you need to practice controlled hyperventilation. This is done by inhaling and exhaling quickly multiple times, before taking that last, big breath. The rush of oxygen to the blood reduces the levels of CO_2 and tricks the brain into thinking that the blood is oxygenated enough, and there's no need to panic.

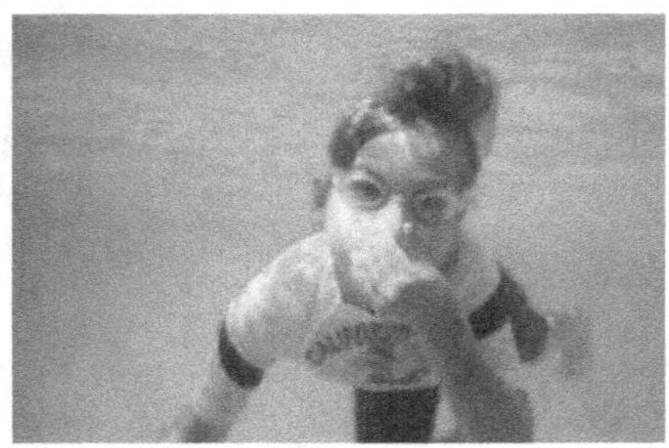

16. Quickly Stop "Pins & Needles."

If you're suffering from the achy feeling of pins and needles in one of your limbs, you can make that feeling go away in a simple manner. If the feeling is in your arms, tilt your head from side to side several times and the tingling sensation will dissipate within 60 seconds. That is because the tingling sensation often occurs due to tension in the nerve endings located in the neck. By relaxing the neck muscles, you ease the strain on those nerve endings. If your legs "fall asleep", on the other hand - get up and walk.

17. Improve Your Short-Term Memory

Professor Candi Heimgartner of the biology department at the University of Idaho, explains that memory processes that occur during sleep are the most effective, so anything you learn before bedtime will be registered better in the long term. This means that if you have a test or a presentation tomorrow, study the main points before you go to sleep.

Ref: http://www.ba-bamail.com/

Short Tips to Keep You in Tip Top Health

Anyone will tell you that nothing is more important than your health, and staying healthy should be your #1 priority. These 25 little tips, tricks, and pieces of advice should help you and those around you to stay healthy.

1. If you feel like eating but are not sure if you're really hungry, ask yourself if you'd like to have an apple. If the answer is 'no', you're most likely bored rather than hungry.

2. Exercising before going to bed makes your muscles burn more calories during the night.

3. Crying releases excess stress hormones and is scientifically proven to ease mental strain.

4. A mid-day nap improves your memory and reduces the chances of developing heart diseases.

5. If you're feeling anxious and stressed, eat a melon. Melons help relieve anxiety and stress, plus they boost your metabolism.

6. Start learning a new language or how to play an instrument. These actions help slow down the brain's aging process.

7. While driving, chew mint or cinnamon-flavored gum. It has been proven to reduce feelings of frustration by 25%, increase your vigilance by 30%, and makes the drive feel 30% shorter.

8. You can 'program' your brain to be happy in a simple way: think of three things you're grateful for every day. Do this for 21 days and you'll notice the change.

9. Skipping a meal can cause you to gain weight. Your body thinks you're going through a famine, which causes it to work in energy-saving mode and makes burning calories more difficult.

10. Listening to music regularly is said to reduce the chances of developing a brain tumor.

11. Drink two cups of cold water before a meal, as this boosts metabolism by up to 30%.

12. If you suffer from headaches or mental stress, lie down next to a wall with your legs elevated and leaning against the wall at a 90-degree angle. Maintain this position for 5 minutes.

13. Running for half an hour a day will help you reduce 0.5kg (1 lb) of fat a week.

14. Drinking a lot of water during the day helps you sleep better at night.

15. Women who walk for an hour each day reduce their chances of getting breast cancer by 15%.

16. Check your toothpaste for an ingredient called "Novamin" – it is the only substance that can repair teeth.

17. Natural pineapple juice is 5 times more effective than cough syrup. It can also prevent baldness, and even the flu.

18. Make an effort to eat a home-cooked meal at least 5 times a week. A recent study found that this may extend your life by a whole decade.

19. If you're trying to quit smoking, try the following method: every time you feel the need to smoke a cigarette, lick a tiny bit of salt. The urge to smoke should pass within a month.

20. A cold shower can help relieve depression and also helps keep your skin and hair healthier.

21. If you've stayed up all night, take a 15-minute nap before sunrise. It will trick your body into thinking it slept enough. (Don't do this too often.)

22. Having a pet reduces stress, improves mental functions and extends your life expectancy.

23. Make an effort to be organized. The more organized you are – the less likely you are to suffer from Alzheimer's.

24. The first day of the week defines your thinking patterns for the week. It's best to exercise during that day, to assure a healthy routine.

25. If you've worn shoes for a long period of time, rub alcohol on your feet. This will help disinfect the regions that are susceptible to fungus

Ref: http://www.ba-bamail.com/

Health Checks Worth Doing on a Regular Basis

Illness is something we as humans are forever dreading, especially since we know some cases can be chronic or life-threatening. The worst part is, we don't realize we're ill until the symptoms become unavoidable. By following the self-checks below you can assure yourself of your body's health - they're quick, easy and definitely worth knowing! You'd be surprised to see what the smallest sign in your body may indicate.

1. **Check your eyes for cholesterol levels**
   A lack of white in your eyes normally indicates that you're tired or hung-over, but surprisingly enough, excess white in your eyes, such as a white line circling your iris, might be indicative of high cholesterol levels. Finding that your eyelids have a flat, yellowish color with velvety patches is also a serious sign. Do not let this symptom go unnoticed and risk getting further complications, such as coronary heart disease, which can lead to heart attacks in the future. See your GP to get your cholesterol checked and treated!

2. **Count your moles to check for skin diseases**
   Moles are generally harmless, but if you find that you have more than 50 moles on your body, take this as a big warning sign, especially if they are multi-colored, growing in size, seem inflamed, or have a ragged edge. If you notice any of these signs in your moles, a good idea would be to regularly keep a record of their development by taking photos so it would be easier for your doctor to inspect them. If your moles also start to redden, become itchy or even bleed, seek medical advice as soon as possible. Such unusual- looking moles may be the cause of a type of skin cancer called malignant melanoma. Take our moles test to see if you know your moles.

3. **Look for signs before you flush the toilet**
   Our excretions can also tell us about the health of our intestines, our digestion and our level of hydration. Every stool color, for instance, indicates different dietary causes or even problems. For example, a yellow color indicates excess fats, due to a malabsorption disorder such as celiac disease. What is most worrying is finding black or red stools, which may signify stomach or intestinal bleeding. These call for prompt medical attention. Urine can also be checked for its color: A pale color signifies good health, whereas a dark yellow color might mean you're dehydrated and need to increase your intake of water. Learn more about what the color of your urine says about your health.

4. **Check your eyebrows for thyroid health**
   If you notice an unusual lack of thickness in your eyebrows, it could be that you are suffering from an underactive thyroid, which means that your thyroid gland is not producing enough hormones. You may need to speak to a doctor, especially if you are also gaining weight and feeling tired and/or depressed. A blood test should easily confirm this problem. If left untreated, it might lead to heart disease, the appearance of goiters, pregnancy complications and other health issues.

5. **Watch your stomach for signs of Ovarian cancer**
   Bloating in your stomach area can have a range of different causes, including menstruation, intolerance to dairy products, eating too fast, constipation, medical side-effects, and a typically common assumption - weight gain. However, did you know this could also be the cause of very serious health conditions? Ovarian cancer is one of them, and its symptoms also include nausea and persistent pain or cramps in the stomach or back. Speak to a doctor if you experience these in a severe way so you can treat it in its early stages. Reduce general stomach bloating by eating more slowly, consuming less carbonated drinks, and avoiding chewing gum and drinking through straws.

6. **Check your breathing by doing some step-ups**
   Have you been feeling more tired than usual after climbing up a flight of stairs? This can also be directly connected to your health. Doing some exercise can both act as a test for yourself and also as practice. Step-ups are mostly recommended because they elevate the heart rate and hence our breathing. For this exercise, you must find a relatively high step (not higher than your hips) and step up and down. Try doing 70 of these in three minutes and then put your fingers on your pulse to check it. If it's over 100 and you're still out of breath 10 minutes after the exercise, then you need to consider exercising more frequently. Lack of exercise can lead to serious diseases such as obesity, breast cancer, diabetes, high blood pressure, and even early death.

7. **Calculate the time you spend sitting down daily**
As we become more technology-dependent, we are adopting more of a sedentary lifestyle. According to the US Women's Health Study, women over 50 who sit for 11 hours a day reduce their life expectancy by 9 years! The consequences for a sedentary lifestyle can be very serious, including deep vein thrombosis, colon cancer, osteoporosis, kidney stones and a Spinal disc herniation (slipped disc). Improve your lifestyle by adding regular physical activity to your routine, at least 2.5 hours a week.

8. **Look out for temperature changes in your body**
Care for your blood vessels' health and circulation by observing the temperature changes in your body, especially in extreme temperature conditions. Excess heat from the sun, stress, and eating very spicy food may cause flushing in the face – particularly redness in the cheeks and nose. This means that the blood vessels are dilating and this may not be a healthy sign, especially if you are a woman between 30 and 55. Cold conditions can be just as dangerous to our body if we aren't prepared for them – frequently experiencing cold feet or hands indicates lack of circulation, which could lead to Raynaud's disease (suffering from excessively reduced blood flow). So, make sure to take the necessary precautions before this becomes a risk!

9. **Inspect your nipples for signs of breast cancer**
A well-known pointer that calls for a professional body check-up is having abnormalities in your nipples. Be on the look-out for inward-facing nipples as this could be a typical sign of breast cancer. If your nipples show any eczema, discharge or bloodstains, take action. Make sure to look out for these signs regularly when showering and find time to do regular exercise, eat plenty of fruit and vegetables, and drink less alcohol to reduce the risk of getting breast cancer.

10. **Examine your nails to look out for fungal infections**
It is rather easy for toenails to get an infection and one of the obvious symptoms of this event is when the nail becomes discolored, thickens, or becomes brittle, causing discomfort in your feet. Keep your feet safe from this by checking them regularly, keeping them clean and dry from excess sweat due to the heat, using shoes that are just right for your feet and not too old, not trimming or picking the skin around the toenails, and avoid walking barefoot in public places. If you do suffer from an infected toenail, seek medical assistance and use antifungal spray or powder to treat it.

Ref: http://www.ba-bamail.com/

18 Incredible Things You Didn't Know About Your Body.

The human body is one of the greatest creations of nature, and one of its most mysterious. There is so much to know and learn about our own bodies, and they keep surprising us each and every day. Here are 18 amazing facts you may have never known about the body you live in

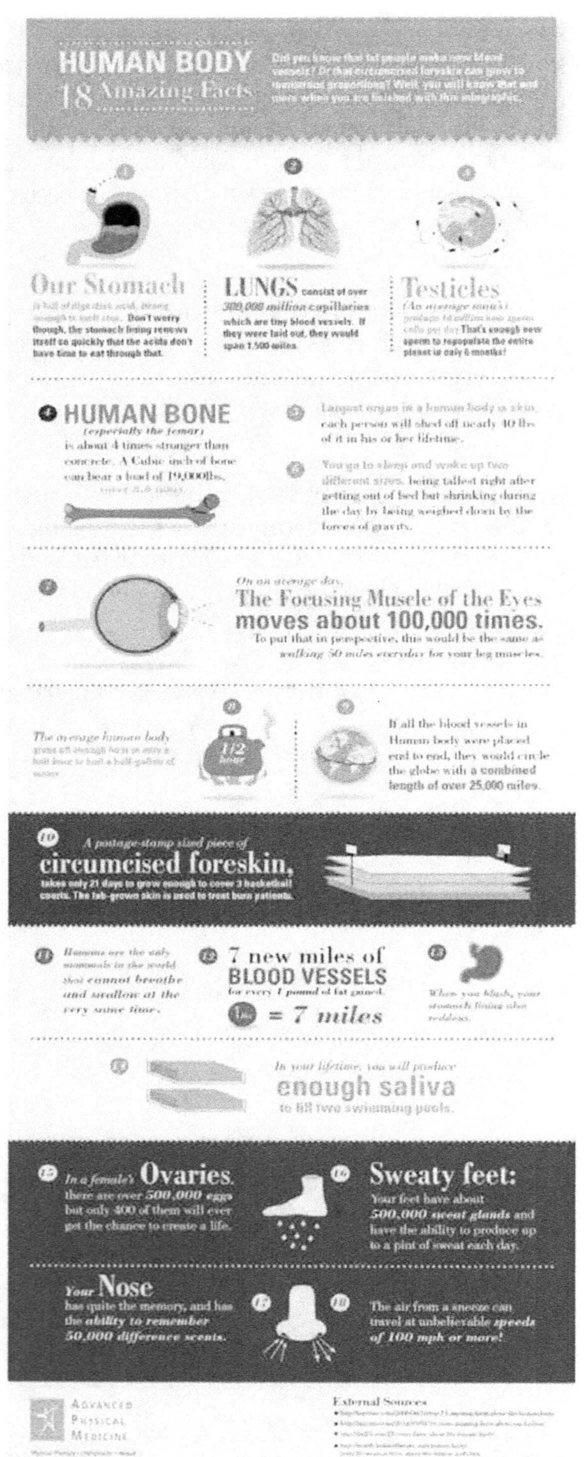

Good to Know - Helpful Pressure Points!

According to ancient oriental beliefs, every organ in the human body has a representative pressure point in the hand and the foot. According to this method, massaging and applying pressure to this point for about 10 minutes should alleviate pain, cure diseases and make us feel much better. Get to know the most important pressure points in the hands and feet:

The Hands

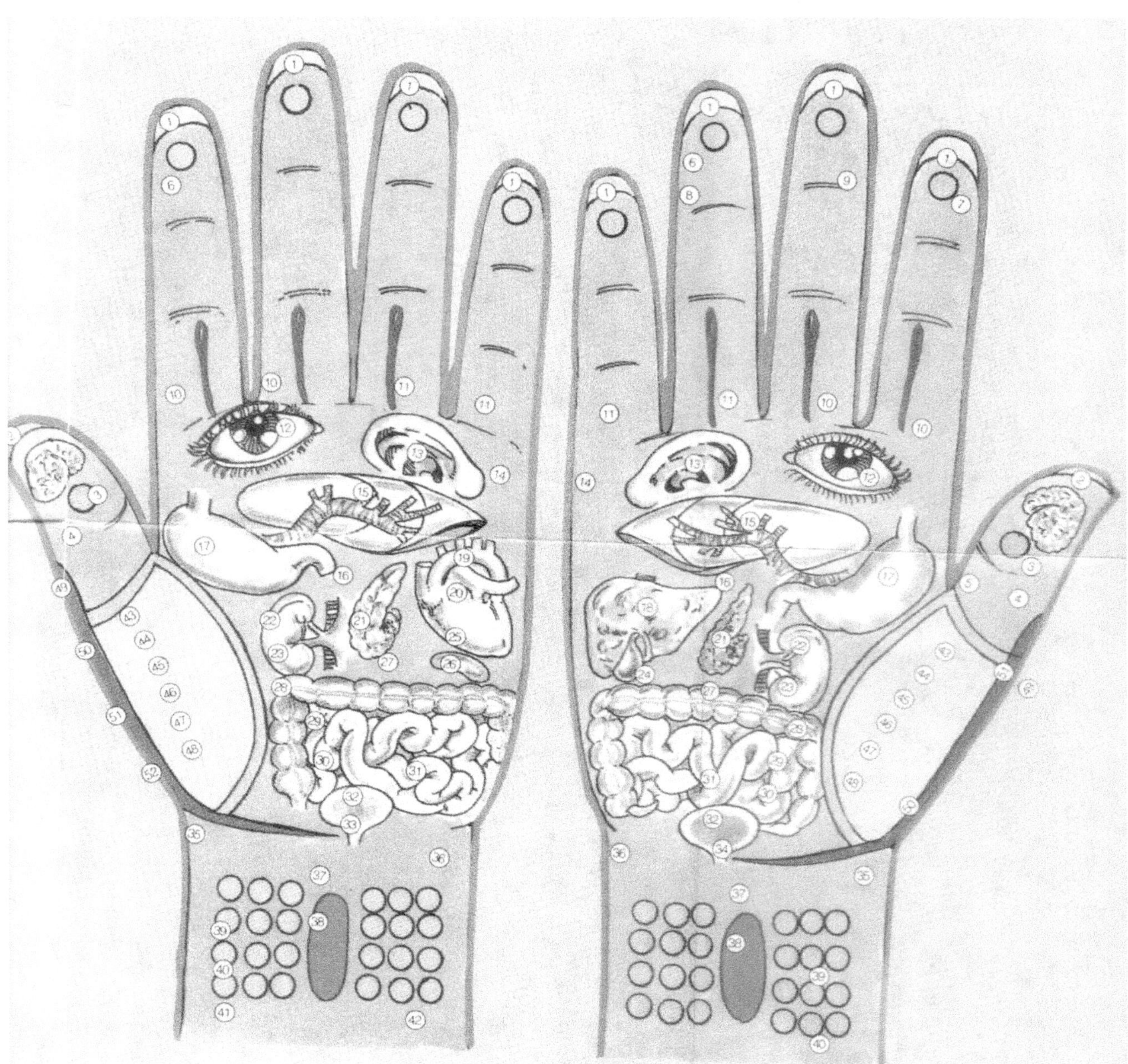

The Feet

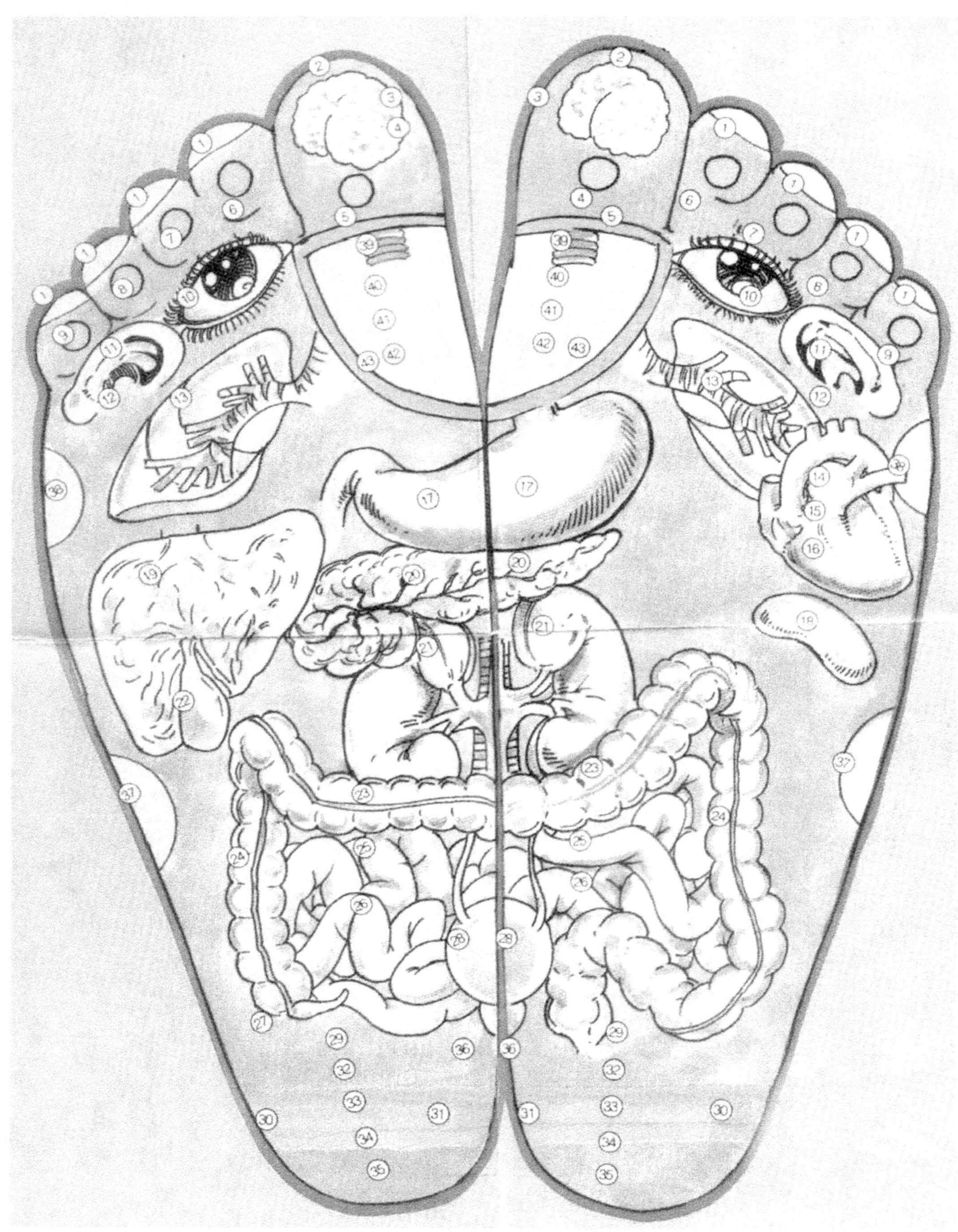

1. Sinusitis

2. Headaches

3. Anxiety

4. Passing Out

5. Insomnia

6. Stimulate Memory

7. Cooling

8. Ear

10. Vision Problems

11. Ear Disease

12. Toothache

13. Lung Disease

14. Heart Disease

15. Blood Flow Disease

16. Hypertension

17. Stomach Disease

18. Spleen Disease

19. Liver Disease

20. Diabetes

21. Kidney Disease

22. Small Intestine

23. Digestive Disorders

24. Large Intestine

25. Bulimia

26. Intestinal Obstruction

27. Appendix

28. Bladder

29. Intestines

30. Infertility

31. Sexual Stimulation

32. Joint Pain

33. Leg Pain

34. Heel Pain

35. Hemorrhoids

36. Back Pain

37. Lower Back Pain

38. Shoulder Pain

39. Right Leg Pain

40. Hormone

41. Weight Loss Deficiency

42. Thyroid Nodules

43. Parathyroid Pain

Ref http//www.ba-bamail.com/

The Healing Fingers

We all use touch for therapy — we touch our chins when we're thinking and clasp our hands together when we're uncomfortable. Even babies suck on their thumbs when they go to sleep. We don't do all of these things for nothing, as each part of our body is connected to a whole system. If we know where to apply pressure in the system, we can overcome various physical and mental symptoms.

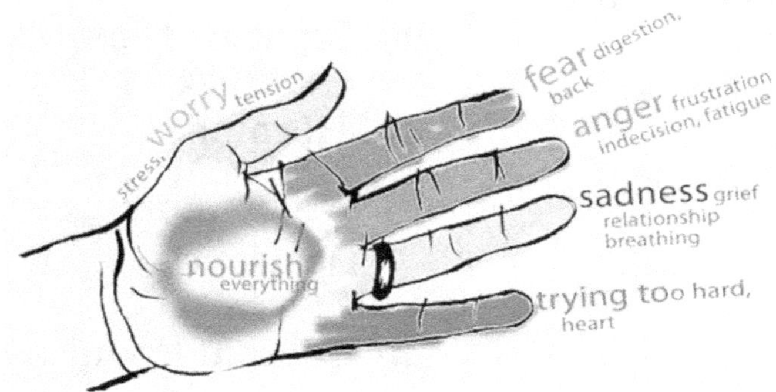

Finger Touch Therapy originates from an ancient Chinese technique, in which every finger relates to different organs and emotions. In a study conducted by the Mercy Cancer Center in the U.S., all of the participants experienced beneficial sensations, including reduced stress and nausea during chemotherapy. Additionally, many patients that reported difficulties sleeping found that by holding their thumb and taking deep breaths, they were able to fall asleep much faster. It is assumed that thumb holding is related to the way babies suck on their thumbs, but either way, both patients and doctors strongly recommend this method. To use this technique, all you have to do is make a fist around the finger that's connected to the sensation or body part you wish to soothe, and slowly apply pressure to it for three to five minutes while breathing deeply. If you want to balance your whole body, simply do it for each finger on both hands.

Thumb

- **Sensations:** Anxiety, worry, and depression
- **Organs:** Stomach and spleen
- **Physical Symptoms:** Stomachaches, headaches, skin problems, and stress

Index Finger

- **Sensations:** Fear, frustration, uncertainty, and confusion
- **Organs:** Kidneys and bladder
- **Physical Symptoms:** Indigestion, discomfort in the arms, elbows and wrists, muscle pains, backaches, teeth related problems, and any type of addiction.

Middle Finger

- **Sensations:** Anger, restlessness, and indecisiveness
- **Organs:** Liver and gall bladder
- **Physical Symptoms:** Eye and vision problems, lethargy, migraines, frontal headaches, period pains, and circulatory system issues.

Ring Finger

- **Sensations:** Sadness, grief, fear of abandonment and rejection, negativity
- **Organs:** Lungs and large intestine
- **Physical Symptoms:** Indigestion, respiratory problems, tinnitus, deep-layer skin problems

Pinky

- **Sensations:** Low self-esteem, judgmental behavior, and stress
- **Organs:** Heart and small intestine
- **Physical Symptoms:** Stomachaches, headaches, skin problems, and stress

Ref: http://www.ba-bamail.com/

The Health Benefits of Different Sleeping Positions

We always hear about how many hours we need to sleep, that a sleep cycle is 1.5 hours and to time our sleep accordingly.

But did you know that your sleeping position can directly help you deal with various pains and irritations?

First, let's have a look at the average human's biological clock so we know when our sleep is most effective:

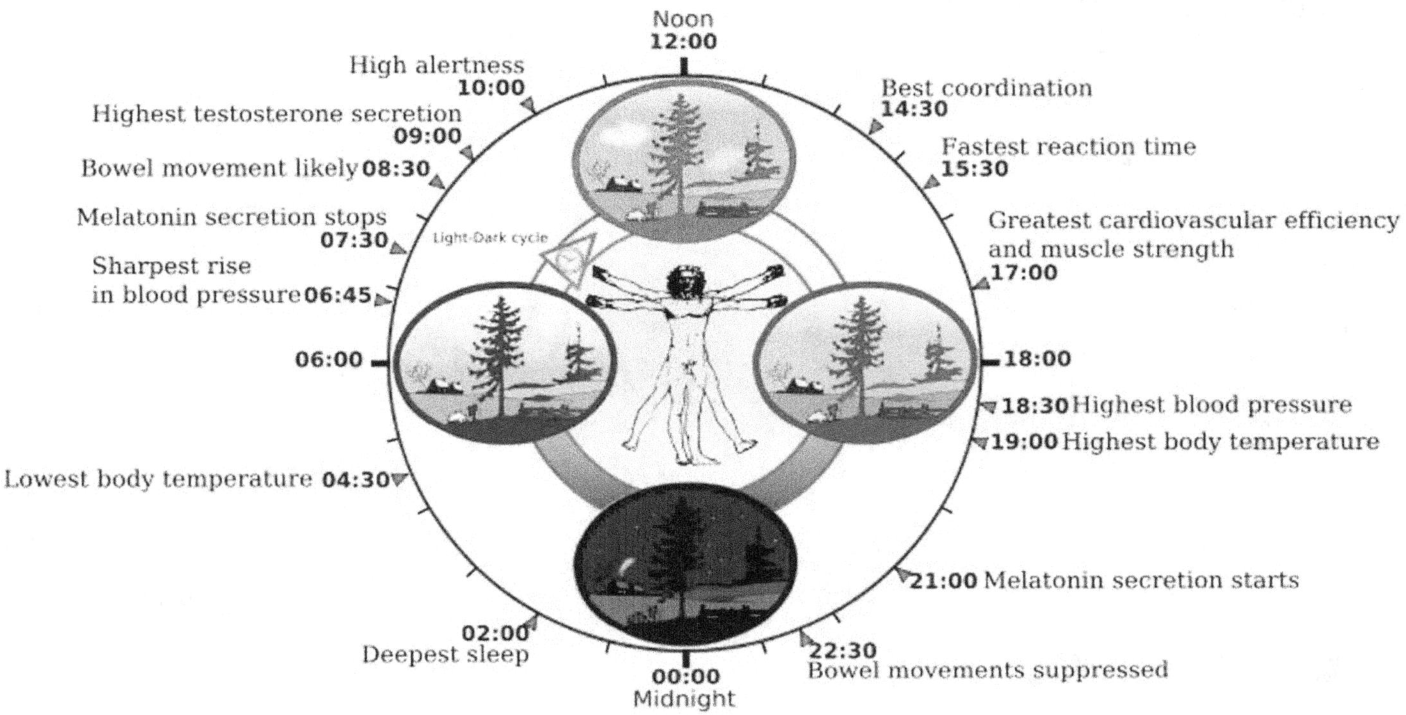

it's important to remember that sleep deprivation is a dangerous thing with very severe consequences:

Wikipedia

Now let's look at the best way to lie down when you go to sleep, according to what bothers you:

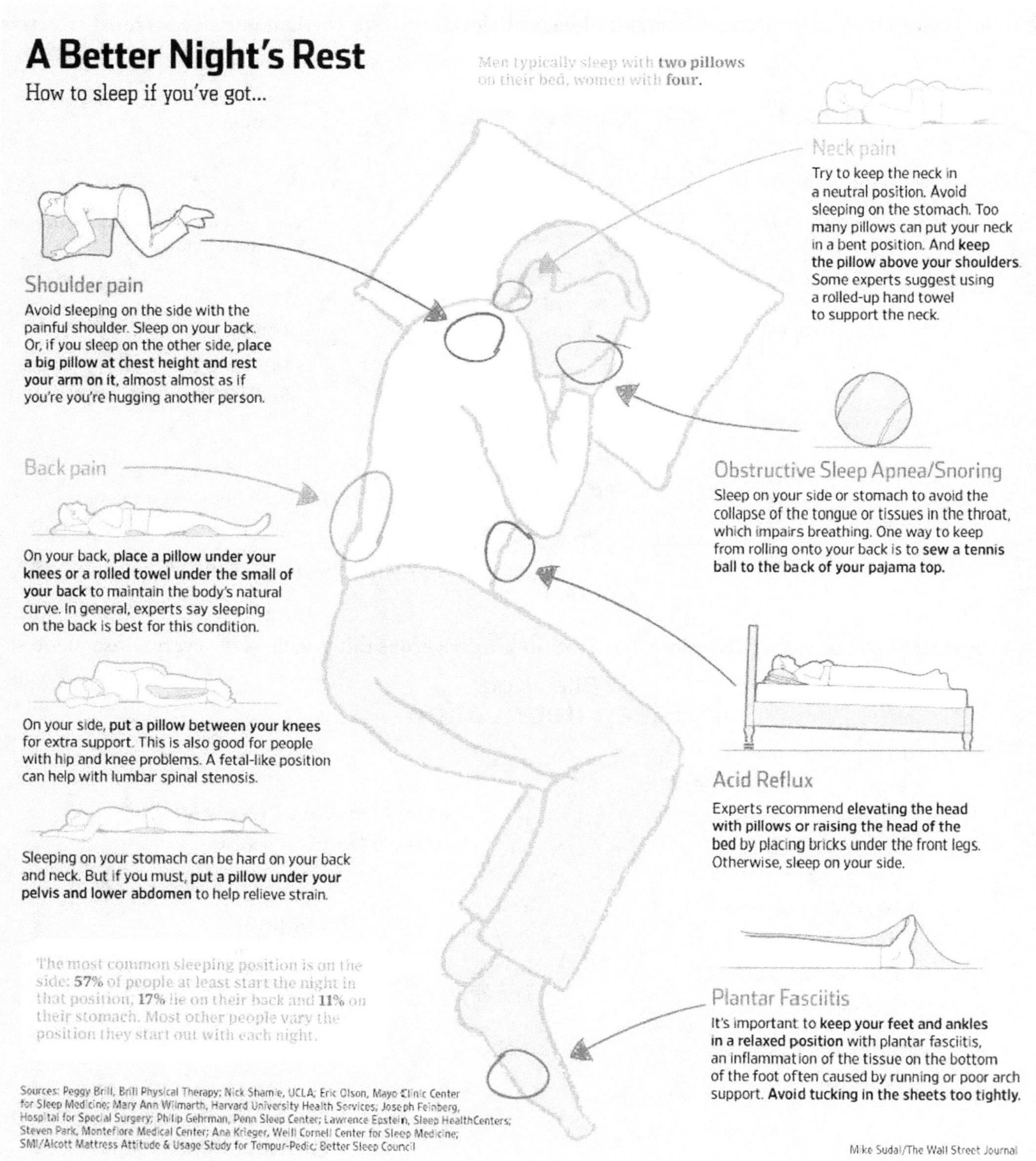

9 Potentially Fatal Medication Mistakes You Should Avoid

The numbers are nothing less than shocking — no less than 1.5 million people are injured or made ill due to medication mistakes, and some 100,000 of those actually end up dying each year. The sad thing is that all these deaths are completely preventable. The answer to avoiding such tragic and unfortunate situations is to protect ourselves from the following medication mistakes:

1. **Confusing two medications with similar names**
   This could happen for a whole variety of reasons, from your doctor's illegible handwriting, to an incorrect input into a pharmacy computer, or even the wrong drug being pulled from the shelf. According to the national Medication Error Reporting Program in the US, similar drug names account for 25 per cent of all reported errors.
   How to avoid it: Ask your doctor to write down what your medication is when he's writing your prescription in addition to the name and dosage. Check the label on your medication when you pick it up from the pharmacy and ensure that the name, dosage and directions for use are the same as on your prescription.

2. **Taking two or more drugs that magnify each other's side effects**
   While it's true that any drug can have side effects, the side effects you experience can be exponentially worse when you combine two or more drugs that interact with each other negatively.
   How to avoid it: Ask your doctor about potential side effects when given a new prescription, and make sure your pharmacy gives you a printout about the medication so that you can review it later. If you see the same side effect listed for more than one medication, make sure you check with your pharmacist or doctor to see if they're safe to take in combination.

3. **Overdosing by combining medications with similar properties**
   It's very easy to end up taking medications that all work in a similar way to each other, even though they may have been prescribed to treat different conditions. For example, the pain and anxiety medications you're taking could both be sedatives, and their combined effect on your body could be toxic.
   How to avoid it: Pay attention to warnings written on the packaging of any over-the-counter medication you may be purchasing, as well as the risks listed in the documentation for prescription. Look out for key words, such as "sleepy", "drowsy", "dizzy", "sedation" and their equivalents.

4. **Taking wrong dosages**
   Medication is prescribed in a variety of units of measure, which are sometimes annotated as abbreviations or symbols. This offers plenty of opportunity for a disaster to happen — all it takes is a misplaced decimal point for 1.0mg to become 10mg. It goes without saying that such a miscalculation can be fatal.
   How to avoid it: If you can't read the dosage of a medication on your prescription, then chances are that a pharmacist or nurse will also have difficulty. Ask the pharmacist to check whether the dosage you've been prescribed by your doctor is within the range that's typical for the particular type of medication. If you're in the hospital, don't be afraid to speak up if you think you're about to receive incorrect medication or an incorrect dosage.

5. **Mixing alcohol with medications**
   Alcohol turns into a deadly poison when mixed with any of a long list of painkillers, sedatives or other medications. In fact, medical experts say it's not safe to drink when taking any kind of medication unless your doctor has explicitly said it is safe to do so
   How to avoid it: It's better to check with your doctor whether it's safe to take the medication you've been prescribed and also drink alcohol. He or she may prescribe you an entirely different medication if you happen to be a heavy drinker. Also check the label on your medication to see if it has any alcohol content.

6. **Double-dosing by taking a brand-name medication and a generic version of it simultaneously** It's quite a common occurrence for patients to get confused and end up with bottles or boxes of a brand- name medication and a generic version of it with a different name. This can result in both being taken simultaneously.
   How to avoid it: Ask your doctor to write down both the brand-name and generic names of the medication you've been prescribed. Also ask him or her to include what the medication is for, its correct dosage, how often and when to take it. You should try and remember these names for future reference. Furthermore, research both brand-name and generic versions of your prescriptions before checking all of your medications, for any duplication.

7. **Eating certain foods that can react dangerously with your medications**

Grape juice is definitely something to avoid when you're taking medication because it acts as an inhibitor for a crucial enzyme that helps the body metabolize it and break it down. This results in an overloaded liver, which can lead to an overdose with potentially fatal consequences. Coffee and iron interactions should also be approached with caution – coffee interferes with iron absorption.

How to avoid it: Ask your doctor about taking your medication without food, as well as whether you can eat certain foods while on the medication. Also alert them to any dietary issues or concerns you may have.

8. **Failing to adjust dosages in the event of liver or kidney function loss**

Impaired liver or kidney function means that your body is less able to rid itself of toxins than when you're completely healthy, and this means that medications could build up in your system at higher-than-intended dosages. A serious (sometimes fatal) mistake that doctors make is not decreasing medication dosages in the event of liver or kidney function loss. While liver and kidney function tests should take place before doctors prescribe certain medications, research has indicated that these tests are not conducted as often as they should be.

How to avoid it: Make sure you check the medications you've been prescribed to see if they mention liver or kidney function. Let your doctor know if you've had a recent liver or kidney screening.

9. **Taking medication that's unsafe for your age**

As you age, your body begins to process medications differently. Drugs that cause side effects such as dementia, dizziness, or high blood pressure are much riskier to take for people over the age of 65.

How to avoid it: The Beers List, which is a list of medications that can no longer be considered safe for people over 65, was first compiled in the early 1990s. Take a copy of this list to your doctor and ask him or her to check all your prescribed medications against it. If you're taking a medication that's considered risky, ask for your doctor to find you a safer alternative.

Ref: http://www.ba-bamail.com/

The Effects of Aging on Your Digestion

As you age, your gastrointestinal tract does too. That means that it is important to monitor the foods you eat not only to maintain a healthy weight, but also to ensure that you are taking the best care of your digestive system. Here are five ways that your digestion can change as you age and tips for taking the best care of yourself and your health.

1. **Chewing**

   As you age, chewing food can become more difficult, especially if you have dentures or poor dentition. You may not think of chewing as part of the digestive process, but it is in fact the first and most important step in taking care of your digestive system. When you chew, you are breaking down the food so that the stomach acid and intestinal enzymes can later break it apart into nutrients to be absorbed into your intestines. In order to avoid choking on your food or slowing down your digestion, make sure to chew your food as thoroughly as possible or to cut up your food into smaller pieces. Also, it is important to continue visiting the dentist on a regular basis, about twice a year to make sure that your mouth is healthy and ready to chew. Taking calcium and vitamin D supplements or getting them through your diet can also help to your digestion and other aspects of your internal health. Women ages 50-70 should get about 1,200 mg of calcium and 600 IUs of vitamin D and men of the same age should get 1,000 mg of calcium and 600 IUs of vitamin D daily.

2. **Swallowing**

   After chewing, the next most important aspect of your digestion is swallowing your food properly. As you age, your esophagus, or the pipe that connects your mouth with your stomach, does not contract like it used to, making it more difficult to swallow larger pieces of food. Indeed, when individuals over 50 need to swallow large pieces of food, it can take 50 to 100 percent longer for the food to make its way to you stomach because your esophagus muscles are out of shape. One of the most common conditions among aging individuals is called gastroesophageal reflux disease (GERD), which can cause pain or a burning sensation in your chest when you digest and even the narrowing of your esophagus. Although there is not cure for a narrowing esophagus, one way to prevent this condition and to maximize your digestion with age is to chew your food slowly and in small pieces and to exercise and maintain a healthy weight. Avoid foods high in fat or sodium, which can worsen the feeling of heart burn or reflux, and if the symptoms still do not subside, it is recommended to visit your doctor for medical treatment.

3. **Your Stomach**

   At the end of your esophagus lies the entry into your stomach called the lower esophageal sphincter. As you age, this ring-like muscle at the opening of the stomach gets weaker, once again contributing to heartburn and acid reflux. The muscle fails to relax properly, which allows acid and sometimes other stomach contents to make their way back up the esophagus pipe It is important that if you have suffered from heartburn or indigestion in the past to take note of the foods that may make you feel that way. Spicy and highly acidic foods are some of the major triggers for this condition, along with citrus fruits and high-fat foods. It helps to eat smaller meals that are low in acid and sodium because this can dramatically decrease your chances for heartburn. Another common condition to watch out for in your stomach is called H. Pylori, or a bacteria on your stomach lining that can cause ulcers or sores in the morning or when your stomach is empty. The infection can be detected through blood tests and endoscopy, a small tube inserted in your mouth that extends down to your stomach. If you discover that you have H. Pylori there is no need to worry because the condition can be treated with a combination of antibiotics and acid-suppressing medications.

4. **Intestines**

   With age, your intestines start to get lazy when it comes to absorbing key nutrients like calcium, vitamins A, B- 12, K and D. This is because the muscle movements get slower and the colon function also changes. As a result, adults from ages 50 and up may experience more constipation and have a greater risk of developing colon cancer or diverticulitis, a condition in which small pouches in the colon become infected. As mentioned above, it is recommended to make up for these missing vitamins either in your diet or with supplements. You can relieve your constipation by increasing your daily fiber intake and decreasing your intake of fatty and high-cholesterol foods. In order to naturally increase your fiber intake, eat more whole grains and try to have a fruit or vegetable with every meal. <u>Here are some great ways to naturally increase your daily fiber intake.</u>

5. **Your Liver**
   You may not know that people ages 60 and over have a greater risk of developing gallstones, or hard crystals that form in the gallbladder when your liver is unable to process the cholesterol and other parts of its bile. Bile is a substance you need to digest fat, which is made by the liver, but is stored in the gallbladder. Your risk for gallstones increases with age because the because the bile duct at the opening of your intestine narrows, forcing the bile to stay in the gallbladder for longer periods of time, which causes it to harden. In order to help prevent the formation of gallstones, which can be painful and often require removal surgeries, it is recommended to strictly control your fat intake so as not to overwhelm your gallbladder. Unfortunately, if you have gallstones you most likely won't experience symptoms, and if you do it is usually a mild pain in the pit of your stomach or the upper right part of your belly. The pain can even spread to your right upper back and shoulder blade. If you experience or have experienced any of these symptoms, it is important to immediately contact your doctor.

Lastly, make sure that you remain in constant consultation with your doctor about your digestive health, and ask for extra blood or breath tests the next time you have a check-up.

Ref: http://www.ba-bamail.com/

Daily Habits You Didn't Know Were Boosting Your Health

Good health doesn't simply come from eating healthy food. Being healthy also has a lot to do with the emotional, physical, and mental states we develop from our lifestyle. We might not have the natural urge to eat healthy when our body needs it, but there are things we unknowingly do to improve our lifestyle. You probably didn't know that singing can prevent a cold, or that chewing gum can make you smarter, or that running barefoot does wonders for your body. Here are a couple of ordinary things you do every day that leave a positive impact on your health and wellbeing.

1. **Watching re-runs - Restores mental energy**
    You might often find yourself watching a re-run of one of your favorite shows, and get the feeling that you're awfully wasting time, even though you'd be, in a way, enjoying it. Well, according to scientists at the University of Buffalo, re-watching shows and movies actually has a calming and re-energizing effect on your brain. The fact that you already know the plot line means that the activity requires minimum mental effort. So if you've just completed a demanding task, which left you feeling drained, consider watching re-runs - an excellent idea to restore your mental energy.

2. **Singing - Prevents a cold**
    We all know that singing can improve our mood significantly. However, here we are not referring to solo singing, but rather to singing with other people, as this activity requires more coordination. Studies have shown that group singing can increase the levels of s-IgA (secretory immunoglobulin A), which is the antibody in saliva that prevents us from contracting bacterial and viral infections. Studies show that people who sing in groups, such as choir singers, have been found to have lower stress levels, as well as better moods - two things that contribute to a healthier immune system.

3. **Laughing with friends - Increases pain tolerance**
    Laughter is the best medicine - but the joy you get from watching a funny show alone might not be as fulfilling as the one you get from being in good company. Laughing, in general, has a lot of benefits, including higher tolerance of pain, due to the release of endorphins (feel-good chemicals) in the brain. However, researchers at Oxford University found that the relief of pain was more effective when they tested people who laughed along with others, rather than people who laughed at comedies alone.

4. **Chewing gum - Sharpens your wits**
    It's not the first time I heard myths about chewing gum, and how it can negatively affect my health. But a group of British researchers have actually found that people who chew gum showed higher accuracy rates and faster reactions than those who don't, after they had been given certain sequences of numbers and were asked to remember them. This basically suggested that gum chewing may be beneficial for the brain, in such a way that it improves cognitive functions such as memory, attention, alertness, and intelligence.

5. **Watching a wall-mounted TV - Eases neck and back pain**
    There's a tendency that wall-mounted TVs are hung above eye-level on a wall, unlike many ordinary standing TVs, which are placed lower. It has been found that such positioning is more comfortable for your head, which would need to be tilted up slightly. According to Scott Bautch (an ergonomics and occupational health expert), this is said to cause less stress on your neck, since watching TV at eye-level automatically tilts the head forward, using 2 or three times more muscle energy as a result.

6. **Sipping on ice water - Diffuses a fight**
    When we're feeling infuriated and are bound to start a fight, we would perhaps think of (or be given) a warm drink to calm us down. In reality, this won't work the way you want it to. If you really want to cool down your angry mood, pour yourself a glass of cold water, a cold slush, smoothie or frozen coffee. Apparently, this will make you more inclined to see someone else's point of view when you're not in the right mood.

7. **Using a cafeteria tray - Encourages healthier eating**
    This news might be rather surprising - but did you know that when you opt for a food tray at the canteen or cafeteria, you are more likely to pick healthy food? At many food places, trays are considered a factor to increased food waste, but according to Cornell University researchers, the use of trays encourages diners to include dishes such as salads, entrées and desserts in their lunch. When you do not use a tray, there's a bigger chance that you leave one of these dishes out - and the first one would probably be a salad!

8. **Walking barefoot - Promotes foot health**

When we look to improve our feet's health, we generally go roundin search for comfortable shoes, which are cushioned andpurposely structured. Although this helps greatly, you might be missing out on one thing - staying barefoot. This might sound odd, but you have no idea how beneficial it is to make the most of your foot's natural physiology, and unfortunately, shoes don't support that. In fact, they sometimes cause stress on certain parts of the feet. So, every now and then, free your feet and spend some time walking or running barefoot, whether indoors or outdoors - there's absolutely no harm in doing so!

H/T: Reader's Digest

Crucial Tips for Protecting Your Bones

Osteoporosis is a disease that damages the bones and makes them brittle and easily breakable. The disease causes a significant decrease in bone density, and this causes the bone to weaken and increases the risk of fractures.

Our bones are always building and breaking down their issue; When the balance between building and breaking is changed, then the bone density goes down. With age, this problem has a horrible way of increasing in occurrence.

Before you are 10 important tips for the treatment and prevention of decreasing bone density:

1. Yes, you guessed it - **Physical activity.**
   Physical activity, besides being the best thing you can do for yourselves, helps the bones become denser by putting pressure on them, which may prevent the disease to begin with. We recommend using weights to strengthen the skeletal muscles.

2. **Increase your calcium intake -**
   Good sources: Green leaves, soy, sardines, broccoli and nuts. Regular bovine milk isn't that good a source of calcium because of its low absorption rate.

3. **Increase your omega 3 intake** - These fatty acids can be found in flaxseeds or fish: Salmon, cod, and halibut - and are essential to keeping your bones strong.

4. **Reduce caffeine and alcohol intake** - Sorry, but coffee and alcohol 'release' calcium from the bones and damage the hormonal balance in the body, which is important to keeping them strong.

5. **Reduce red meat** - Seems like we're taking all the fun out of lunch, but eating red meat actually reduces the absorption of calcium in the body.

6. **No smoking** - Cigarette smoke damages bone density.

7. **Eat nuts and almonds** - These contain magnesium which is essential to the process of absorbing calcium.

8. **Get at least 15 minutes of sun exposure a day** - Exposing your skin to the sun a few minutes a day is the best way of getting your vitamin D, which functions as a sort of glue and helps keep the bone density up.

9. **Eat sunflower seeds** - These contain zinc, a key mineral for maintaining strong bones.

10. **Make sure you're not lacking in these elements**, and take according to professional opinion: Boron, Silicone, vitamin C, vitamin D, calcium, magnesium, vitamin B12, vitamin B6 and folic acid.

Ref: http://www.ba-bamail.com/

18 Reasons to Keep Hydrogen Peroxide at Home

Hydrogen Peroxide is an active agent material composed of nothing more than water and oxygen. The oxidation process of this material is incredibly good at killing disease organisms, and HP is considered one of the world's safest, all natural, sanitizer. It literally 'burns' micro-organisms by oxidation. However, this material has so many other uses, it was really hard to pick only the best or most useful ones to share with you. So, I've done my best to highlight some of the nifty things you can do with it. **Tip:** Make sure to only use the 3% solution for most of these items, and do not use it for internal purposes (do not swallow). Higher strength solutions such as 30% may cause damage if ingested.

1. **Whiten your clothes with HP instead of bleach**
   By adding a cup of HP to the white clothes in your laundry, you will see a marked improvement in how white they are. This is a great way of getting rid of really incessant stains such as blood or wine. For blood, just pour directly on the spot, wait a minute, and then rub and rinse under cold water.

2. **Boosting your immune system**
   Your body makes its own HP to battle infections. Our white blood cells, also known as Leukocytes, are the cells responsible for fighting disease, viruses and infections, and some of them produce HP as their first form of attack and defense from toxins, infections, viruses, parasites and alike.

3. **Making a rejuvenating detox bath**
   Take 2 quarts of 3% HP and pour it into a tub of warm water. Get in and enjoy a good soak for about 30 minutes, adding hot water as needed. This will help skin blemishes, detox your body and rejuvenate you in a way you haven't felt before.

4. **Treating foot fungus**
   To use HP to cure your foot fungus, make a mixture of 50% HP and 50% water, and use a spray bottle to spritz the infected area (especially the toes) every night. Let it dry naturally.

5. **Treating Yeast Infections**
   Add 2 caps or 2 tablespoons of 3% HP to warm, distilled water once or twice a week and use it to treat the problematic area.

6. **Cleaning your toothbrush and other hygienic tools**
   There are many objects we use that need to be kept clean and sanitized, such as your tooth brush, or your child's retainer. Use a small amount of HP and dilute it with cold water to make a cleansing brew that will make sure they are clean and germ free.

7. **Treating exterior Infections**
   If you have a cut that is infected, soak it in 3% HP for about 5-10 minutes, several times a day. HP is extremely good for treating infections, and you can also pour half a bottle of it in your bath to get rid of fungus, boils or any other skin infections.

   Note: Do not leave on open wounds for a long time, use the solution and then wipe it off. Over time, HP can do tissue damage to open wounds if left on them for too long.

8. **Killing mite infections**
   Patients have reported that spraying HP on skin infected by tiny mites that bite and cause irritation, effectively kills them with incredible efficiency. Spray the area a few times, and wait a few minutes between applications.

9. **Taking care of your Sinus Infection** Add a tablespoon of 3% HP to 1 cup of (non-chlorinated) water, and use it as a nasal spray. You may have to adjust the amount of HP used according to the severity of the problem. Start with just the 1 spoon first.

10. **Using as mouthwash and for tooth care**
    Take a capful or a tablespoon of 3% HP and hold it in your mouth for 10 minutes, once a day. **Do not swallow**, just spit it out. This will not only get rid and prevent canker sores, but will also whiten your teeth. It will also help in the event of a bad toothache you can't treat right away. 10 minutes several times a day will lessen the pain to a more manageable level. It also makes for a great and inexpensive mouth wash. Again, make sure not to swallow and rinse your mouth with regular water after use.

11. **Lighten the color of your hair**
HP is a bleaching agent and can be used to lighten your hair. Take a bottle of 3% HP and dilute some with water (50/50). Take a shower and, while the hair is still wet, spray it with the solution, then comb it through. It won't look like a burnt blonde color, but a more natural highlight for those with light brown, reddish or dirty blond hair. It is also a gradual change so you won't have a drastic new look on your hands.

12. **Clean your contact lenses**
As a great disinfectant, due to its remarkable skill in breaking down the proteins that build up on the lens, HP can not only clean contact lenses, but will also increase the level of comfort if you have sensitive eyes, removing those little biological irritants that most solutions don't clean.

13. **Boosting your dishwasher**
Add about 2 oz. (60 ml) of 3% HP to your regular formula, and see how much cleaner the dishes are.

14. **Make sure your cooking surfaces are disease free**
Fill a spray bottle with the 50/50 solution we've talked about (50% water 50% HP) and use it to spray your wooden cutting boards and cooking areas after you are done, to kill salmonella or any other bacteria that might be growing there. To be extra sure, use vinegar after the HP.

15. **Make a cheap and effective disinfectant**
Make a cheap and very effective disinfectant agent that is non-toxic and can be used to disinfect fruits, vegetables, pet bowls, equipment and alike. Combining vinegar and HP has been proven in several studies to kill pretty much all Salmonella, Shigella, and E. coli bacteria. For this, prepare TWO spray bottles. Don't mix these two together. One will contain regular vinegar and the other regular Hydrogen peroxide.

(Tip: *Light is bad for peroxide, rending it inactive. So the best thing will be to keep it covered and in the bottle*).

16. **Treating Mold**
If you have those little spots appearing on your walls, probably from water damage, taking care of them is better done sooner than later, or they can get toxic and dangerous. Clean them with HP a few times a day to kill them off.

17. **Helping sprouting seeds**
If you're trying to get a seed to grow stronger, add an ounce (30 ml) of 3% HP to 1 pint of water and let the seeds soak in it overnight. Every time you rinse the seeds, add the same amount of HP. They will grow faster and healthier.

18. **Preparing Vegetables**
Wash or soak vegetables in a full sink of cold water mixed with a 1/4 cup of 3% HP. Thin-skinned vegetables (such as lettuce) should soak for about 20 minutes, while thicker-skinned ones (such as cucumbers) can soak for about 30 minutes. Then drain, dry and refrigerate. This will not only kill all bacteria and neutralize chemicals, but will also make sure they keep fresh in the refrigerator for longer.

Ref: http://www.ba-bamail.com/

Your Ultimate Guide to Discovering Your Tummy Type

Not all sagging stomachs are the same. They come in different shapes and sizes and appear for all sorts of reasons. Sagging stomachs may be caused by alcohol or stress, feeling bloated, thyroid problems and more. Yet while a tummy caused by wine sticks out mainly at the front, a bloated stomach feels hard to touch. The guide below will help you determine what your tummy type is, and how to shrink its size.

1. Wine tummy

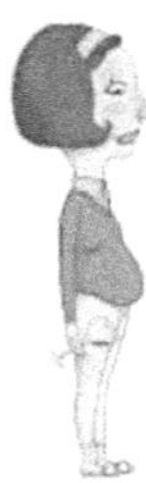

Appearance: While there is less weight gain around your hips and bottom, a wine tummy mainly sticks out at the front. Its appearance resembles that of a pot belly.
The layer of fat stretches from your stomach to your pelvis and may also seep between the vital organs located in this area: the intestines, bowel and liver. Fat gathers in this area because the fat cells are very sensitive to the effects of insulin (a hormone that dictates how much fat is stored in the body). So, when the sugars from booze are released into the body, insulin is released, telling the body to store it as fat within this deep layer.
Cause: Binge drinking and alcohol. Eating too many refined carbohydrates is also a cause.
Studies show that women who drink more than 12 units in a single sitting gain an extra 4 inches around their waist. In another study conducted on 57,000 people by the Center for Alcohol Research in Denmark, heavier drinkers are more likely to develop a rounded, apple-shaped tummy than those who drink in moderation.
Shed the weight: Watch the calories as you drink.
Alcohol typically slows down metabolism by up to 70%. Generally, this effect does not last long, however, if it becomes a habit, it can make you pack on the pounds, primarily at the waist. Monitor the calories you drink just as much as the ones you eat - doing so may help you resist a third or fourth glass. Bear in mind that a large 250ml glass of wine is equivalent to a 228 calorie ice-cream. Another noteworthy point is that alcohol stimulates appetite, encouraging you to eat more. Consequently, that weight gain will be stored deep inside the body.

2. Bloated tummy

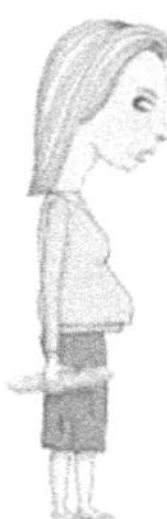

Appearance: A bloated tummy predominantly sticks out at the front. The skin feels hard to touch, almost as if there's an inflated balloon deep inside.
You'll likely start off with a flat tummy at the start of your day, which tends to expand as time goes on, especially after a meal. Nevertheless, no matter how big your tummy gets, your weight will remain the same on the scale.
Cause: A buildup of wind.
Food gets broken down as it travels through the intestines. The bacteria that breaks down the food creates six to eight liters of gas as a by-product. But if the bacteria has difficulty breaking down certain foods, it will start to ferment, creating more wind. Consequently, it starts to push the abdominal wall outwards. Furthermore, constipation and eating too much may also be a cause. And as a result, too much food in the stomach can cause bloating.
Shed the weight: Refrain from eating foods that trigger bloating.
Foods that trigger bloating may be harder for the body to digest, in which case it is best to avoid foods such as artificial sweeteners, wheat, garlic and onions. Some fruit like cherries and plums, as well as certain vegetables including artichokes, beetroot and mushrooms, should also be avoided. A lactose-free diet can also help reduce a bloated stomach.

3. Stress tummy

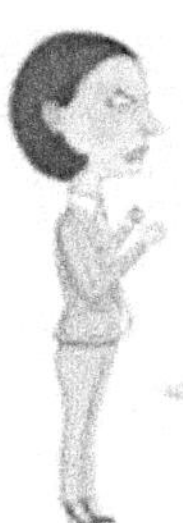

<u>Appearance</u>: **If your tummy bulge is caused by stress, it sticks out from the front, but appears softer and has a saggy appearance, more than that of a pot belly.**
It tends to start under the bust, forming a soft roll which hangs over your waistband.
<u>Cause</u>: **A continuous state of stress.**
When we feel stressed, the fight-or-flight hormone known as cortisol releases sugar into the bloodstream, giving the body energy to escape or defend itself. So, unless you use up this energy (as your body is expecting you to), the energy is simply re-deposited as fat.
<u>Shed the weight</u>: **Engage in relaxation techniques.**
Manage your stress levels with relaxation techniques such as deep-breathing and meditation. A good night's sleep is essential as it encourages the body to no longer feel as though it has to prepare for an attack. Eating small portions and slow-release carbohydrates, like oats and legumes, can also help maintain your stress levels.

4. Pear tummy

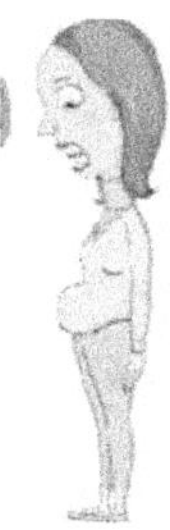

<u>Appearance</u>: **A slim waist, with a roll of fat around your bikini line.**
Aside from fat around your bikini line, women with a pear tummy generally have a bigger bottom and larger hips, creating a pear-shaped look.
<u>Cause</u>: **Female sex hormones, particularly estrogen.**
Some women suffer from estrogen dominance, which may be genetic or triggered by other issues causing an imbalance in female sex hormones. It may also be caused by fibroids - benign tumors of muscular tissue which grow inside the womb. Women may also be exposed to too much estrogen because they ingest high levels of synthetic versions of the hormone from farmed meat, water or residues from chemicals in plastics and water. This type of tummy fat is especially common in women aged 30 to 50. Unless a woman is on hormone replacement therapy, she will likely lose the fat on her hips and thighs, leaving her looking more apple-shaped than pear.
<u>Shed the weight</u>: **Avoid foods high in saturated fats, which have been linked to higher levels of estrogen.**
Opt for a diet high in easy-to-digest fiber, like seeds and green leafy vegetables. These types of food help bind themselves to the extra estrogen in the digestive tract, removing it from the body.

5. Mummy tummy

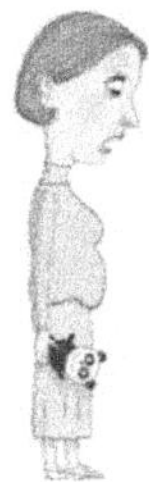

<u>Appearance</u>: **Your tummy area will lack tone and have a saggy-looking appearance.** A mummy tummy becomes apparent three months or more after you've given birth.

Cause: A weak abdominal wall.

During pregnancy and birth, the abdominal muscles divide, enabling your uterus and tummy to expand. Once you have given birth, the two sides of your six-pack muscles should naturally knit back together. If not, you are left with a bulge. This is caused by a weak abdominal wall, that cannot hold in the contents of your stomach and intestines.

Shed the weight: Seek help from a physiotherapist.

A physiotherapist can teach you exercises to help knit your muscles back in place. Pelvic floor exercises will also help strengthen the muscles from within. Yoga poses, like plank pose, are especially useful.

6. **Thyroid tummy**

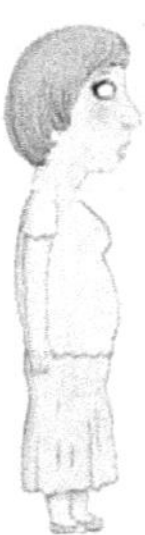

Appearance: Your whole body is big, including your arms and legs.

Cause: Hypothyroidism

A butterfly- shaped gland in the neck produces a hormone called throxine, which controls how fast you process calories in food. However, women who suffer from hypothyroidism make less of this hormone. Women who suffer from hypothyroidism do not burn up all the calories consumed, consequently the extra calories are stored, depositing all over the body as fat. Its exact cause is unknown, however it is believed to be caused by the aging process.

Shed the weight: Eating foods rich in iodine.

Prior to seeking treatment it is important to get proper diagnosis, as hypothyroidism is often confused with mid-life weight gain. Inadequate levels of thyroxine also cause tiredness, constipation and cold feet - all of which contribute to a slower metabolism. Natural treatment includes eating foods rich in iodine, which help support the thyroid, like shellfish, seafood and dark leafy green vegetables. Alternatively, treatment may also include drugs containing a synthetic version of the hormone, to top up levels.

Ref: http://www.ba-bamail.com/

15 Habits that Damage Our Healthy Kidneys

It's hard to notice when we do our kidneys harm. Even if 80% damaged, kidneys can still do their job, and so we rarely realize they're on their last leg. Often, even common daily habits can cause your kidneys continual damage, and when you finally discover something's wrong, it's too late.

Our kidneys are incredible organs that work very hard. By themselves, they absorb minerals and nutrients, produce hormones, act as a filter for toxins in our blood, produce our urine and maintain a normal acid to alkaline ratio. We cannot live without our kidneys functioning properly. The Chinese, for example, have looked at the kidneys as a site of essential life force for centuries.

If you're serious about looking after yourself, then taking care of your kidneys should be one of your primary concerns. If you want to make sure your kidneys thrive and continue to serve you in the coming years ahead, here's a helpful list of habits you should definitely avoid:

1. **Drinking Soda**
   A study conducted on employees working at Osaka University in Japan found that drinking 2 or more soda drinks a day (either diet or regular) may well be connected to a higher risk of kidney disease. The study included 12,000 people, and those who drank larger quantities of soda were found to have protein in their urine, which is one of the first signs of kidney damage. However, early detection can reverse the disease with proper treatment.

2. **A Deficiency in Vitamin B6**
   The healthy function of our kidneys also depends on a healthy diet, especially one that contains certain nutrients. According to a study carried out at the University of Maryland, a vitamin B6 deficiency increases the risk of the formation of kidney stones. For healthy kidney function, a person should have at least 1.3 milligrams of vitamin B6 in their food every day. The best sources for this vitamin are fish, beef liver, potatoes, starchy vegetables, chickpeas and non-citrus fruits.

3. **Smoking**
   Perhaps not surprisingly, smoking has been linked to atherosclerosis - the narrowing and hardening of blood vessels - which influences the blood supply going to all the major organs, including the kidneys. According to a study published in *Clinical Pharmacology and Therapeutics*, just smoking 2 cigarettes a day is enough to double the number of endothelial cells (the cells that line our blood vessel walls) present in your bloodstream. This is a sign of arterial damage. In addition, the *Journal of the American Society of Nephrology* references a number of different studies conducted in the last decade that link smoking to decreased kidney function.

4. **Lack of Exercise**
   Another good way of protecting your kidneys is to get some exercise. A comprehensive study published in 2013 in the *Journal of the American Society of Nephrology* found that postmenopausal women who exercised had a striking 31% less risk of developing kidney stones.

5. **Magnesium Deficiency**
   Magnesium is what helps our body to properly absorb and assimilate calcium. If we don't get enough magnesium, we get overloaded in calcium and, once again, develop kidney stones. To prevent this from happening, add some leafy vegetables, seeds, nuts or beans to your diet. Another good source of magnesium is fresh avocados.

6. **Disrupted Sleep**
   I just love a good night's sleep and, as it turns out, so do my kidneys. According to *Science Daily*, a chronic disruption in our sleep can cause kidney disease. According to Dr. Michael Sole, Cardiologist and Professor of Medicine and Physiology at the University of Toronto, kidney tissues get renewed during the night while we're sleeping, so when we can't sleep without constant interruptions, our kidneys suffer direct damage.

7. **Not Drinking Enough Water**
   One of the most important things for our kidneys is for them to get hydrated enough to perform their functions. If we don't get enough water in our system, toxins start accumulating in our blood because there isn't enough fluid to take them through the kidneys. The National Kidney Foundation recommends drinking at least 10-12 glasses of water every day. An easy way to check if you're drinking enough is to make sure your urine is a light color or clear. If it's dark, you're not drinking enough. You can check the color of your urine with this helpful guide.

8. **Not Emptying Your Bladder Fast Enough**

When you hear the call to pee, you should listen to it. Obviously, we're not always in the right situation to pee right when the need arises, but if you 'hold it in' on a regular basis, it will increase the pressure of urine on your kidneys, which can lead to renal failure or incontinence.

9. **Having Too Much Sodium in Our Diet**

Salt is an important nutrient, but it can cause a disaster when taken in excessive amounts. Over-consumption of sodium will raise your blood pressure and put a lot of strain on your kidneys. We recommend limiting yourselves to no more than 5.8 grams (0.2 ounces) of salt per day. So put down that salt shaker!

10. **Consuming Too Much Caffeine**

We usually drink more caffeine than we think we do. It's in coffee, tea, soft drinks and sodas - before you know it, your body is full of caffeine, which causes your blood pressure to shoot through the roof, and your kidneys to suffer damage.

11. **Abusing Pain-Killers**

Many of us have a daily routine of taking medications. When we suffer from pain, our first reaction is usually to swallow a pill. They do help the pain, but you should think twice before taking too many. All pharmaceutical drugs have side effects, and many of them cause kidney or liver damage. Check out some natural painkillers you can find or make at home. That said, some drugs SHOULD be taken, which brings us to my next point...

12. **Not Taking Certain Drugs You Need**

If you suffer from high blood pressure and/or type 2 diabetes, two very common conditions these days, you will probably also suffer kidney damage. Don't leave these conditions untreated - take your daily meds to reduce your blood pressure and control your insulin levels. Without them, you're almost guaranteed to suffer kidney damage.

13. **Consuming Too Much Protein**

According to a study conducted at Harvard University, an overdose of protein in our diet can cause our kidneys damage. When we digest protein, our body produces a byproduct - ammonia. Ammonia is a toxin that your already hardworking kidneys need to neutralize. This means that the more protein we consume, the harder we make our kidneys work, which can eventually lead to kidney failure.

14. **Not Treating Common Infections**

Sometimes, we all get lazy and ignore a simple cold or a flu, which can push our body to the brink of exhaustion. Studies have shown, however, that people who do not rest or treat their infections often end up with kidney disease.

15. **Consuming Too Much Alcohol**

Now this is a no-brainer. The toxins in alcohol not only damage the liver, like many believe, but they are also something your kidneys simply hate to deal with. According to Kidney Health Australia and the American Kidney Fund, one good way of avoiding kidney failure is drinking alcohol in moderation.

http://www.ba-bamail.com/

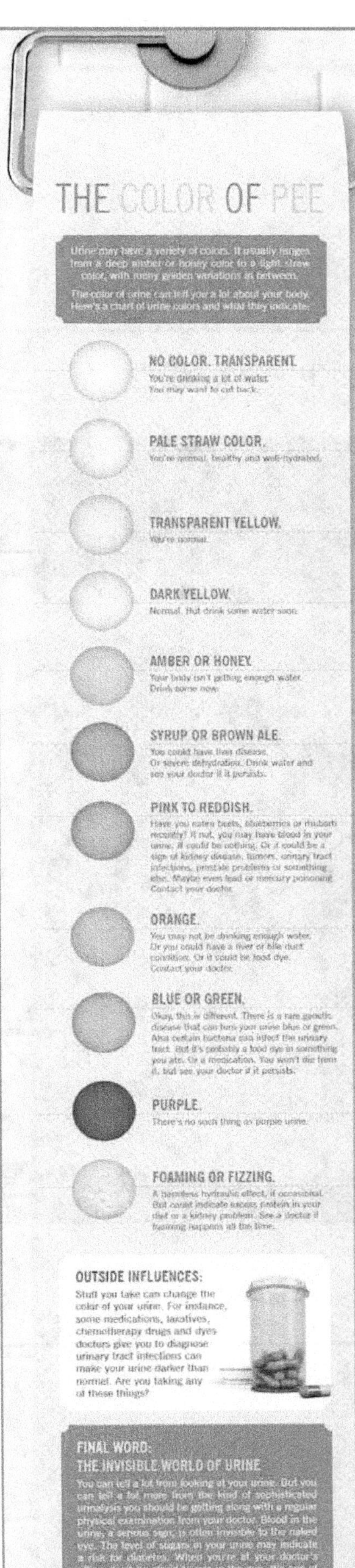

THE COLOR OF PEE

Urine may have a variety of colors. It usually ranges from a deep amber or honey color to a light straw color, with many golden variations in between.

The color of urine can tell you a lot about your body. Here's a chart of urine colors and what they indicate:

NO COLOR. TRANSPARENT.
You're drinking a lot of water. You may want to cut back.

PALE STRAW COLOR.
You're normal, healthy and well-hydrated.

TRANSPARENT YELLOW.
You're normal.

DARK YELLOW.
Normal. But drink some water soon.

AMBER OR HONEY.
Your body isn't getting enough water. Drink some now.

SYRUP OR BROWN ALE.
You could have liver disease. Or severe dehydration. Drink water and see your doctor if it persists.

PINK TO REDDISH.
Have you eaten beets, blueberries or rhubarb recently? If not, you may have blood in your urine. It could be nothing. Or it could be a sign of kidney disease, tumors, urinary tract infections, prostate problems or something else. Maybe even lead or mercury poisoning. Contact your doctor.

ORANGE.
You may not be drinking enough water. Or you could have a liver or bile duct condition. Or it could be food dye. Contact your doctor.

BLUE OR GREEN.
Okay, this is different. There is a rare genetic disease that can turn your urine blue or green. Also certain bacteria can infect the urinary tract. But it's probably a food dye in something you ate. Or a medication. You won't die from it, but see your doctor if it persists.

PURPLE.
There's no such thing as purple urine.

FOAMING OR FIZZING.
A harmless hydraulic effect, if occasional. But could indicate excess protein in your diet or a kidney problem. See a doctor if foaming happens all the time.

OUTSIDE INFLUENCES:
Stuff you take can change the color of your urine. For instance, some medications, laxatives, chemotherapy drugs and dyes doctors give you to diagnose urinary tract infections can make your urine darker than normal. Are you taking any of these things?

FINAL WORD:
THE INVISIBLE WORLD OF URINE
You can tell a lot from looking at your urine. But you can tell a lot more from the kind of sophisticated urinalysis you should be getting along with a regular physical examination from your doctor. Blood in the urine, a serious sign, is often invisible to the naked eye. The level of sugars in your urine may indicate a risk for diabetes. When you're at your doctor's office, don't be afraid to pee in the cup. It's one of the best things you can do for your health.

Food

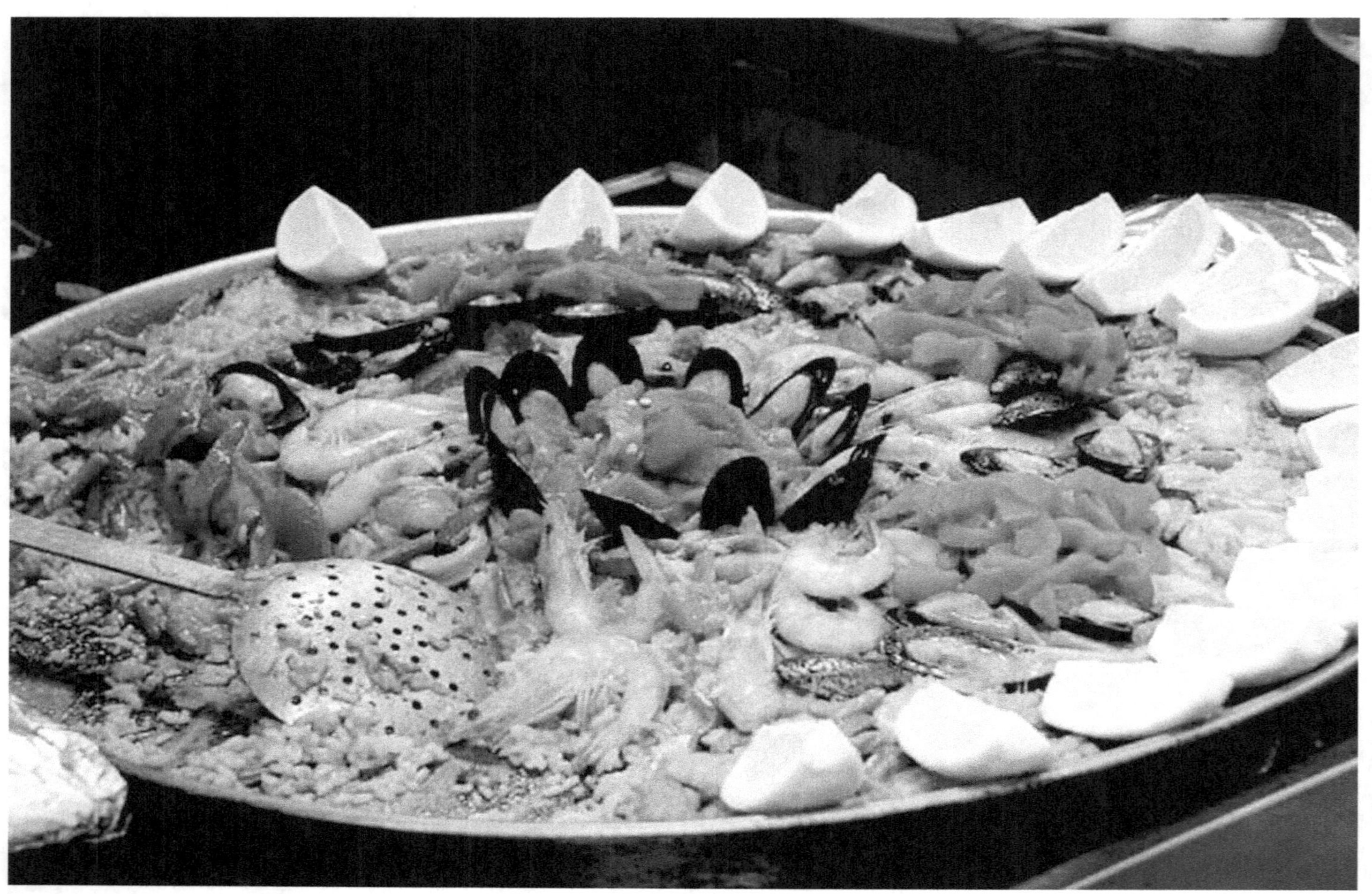

A-Z Sunnah Foods of the Prophet (s.a.w.s.)

Aniseed (anisun)--Among its many properties, the seed of anise soothes internal pains, increases menstrual flow, promotes secretion of milk and semen, and dissolves intestinal gas. It may be applied in tea form to the eyes to strengthen eyesight. In nature, snakes coming out of winter hibernation seek out the anise plant and rub their eyes against it, because their vision becomes weak over winter.

Apple (tuffah)--Sour apples are more cooling than sweet ones. It is claimed that apples strengthen the heart.

Asparagus (hiyawn)--Hot and moist, asparagus opens obstructions of the kidneys and eases childbirth. It is said that asparagus will kill dogs that eat it.

Banana (mawz)--Hot in the first degree, banana has little use as a food, except for people with a very cold intemperament, who should eat it with honey.

Barley (sha'ir)--Barley ranks below only wheat as a desirable food. It is the first recommendation for hot intemperament diseases. Barley is soaked in water, which is drunk for coughs and sore throats. The Prophet (s.a.w.s.) always gave a soup made from barley to anyone suffering from the pain of fever.

Basil, Sweet (rayhan)--Smelling basil strengthens the heart. Sleep is promoted by rubbing the head with basil and water

Bread (khubz)--The best bread is made of the finest whole grain flours and is baked in a circular stone oven. Bread should be allowed to cool somewhat before being eaten, or it will make one excessively thirsty. Stale bread clogs the bowels. Bread containing substantial bran is digested quickly, but is very nourishing. The softer the bread, the easier the digestion and the greater the nourishment. Bread crumbs produce gas. Breads made from barley and pea flours are slow to be digested and must have salt added to them. Said the Prophet (s.a.w.s.): "Do not cut bread with a knife, but give it due honor by breaking it with the hands, for Allah has honored it."

Butter (zubdah)--Butter is mildly hot and moist. Useful to alleviate constipation, butter is also mixed with honey and dates to make a food that removes the food cravings of pregnant women.

Cauliflower (qunnabit)--This vegetable is hard to digest, and it is said to harm the vision.

Chamomile (babunaj)--Hot in the first degree, chamomile is mild. Its main use is to promote urination and menstrual flow.

Carrot (jazar)--Sexual urges arise from eating carrot, which is hot in the second degree. It also is used to increase menstrual flow and urination.

Coconut (narjil darja'i)---The best type is very white, which is hot and moist. The nature of coconut is that it increases sexual powers and relieves pain in the back.

Coffee Bean (qahwah)--Coffee is a corrective for dysentery, relieves thirst, and is said to produce wisdom. It should be used sparingly.

Coriander Seed (habb al-suda)--The most respected books of traditions state that the Prophet (s.a.w.s.) said, "Make yours the seeds of coriander, for it is a cure of all diseases except swelling [cancer], and that is a fatal disease." It is also reported that Allah informed the Prophet, "She has been given every-thing." And then Allah revealed that "she" is coriander. Coriander alleviates flatulence and resolves fevers. It is effective in the treatment of leukoderma, and it opens the subtlest networks of the veins. Excess moisture in the body is dried up by coriander, and it increases milk flow, urine, and menses. It is particularly useful when a person has a cold. The oil of coriander is a treatment for baldness and scalp problems, and prevents gray hair. The smoke of the burning seeds is an insect repellent.

Chicken (dajaj)--Light on the stomach and easy to digest, chicken is the best of fowl meats. It corrects and balances all the essences, is a food that is good for the brain, and improves the complexion. However, overconsumption of chicken leads to gout. The best chicken is a hen that has never laid an egg.

Cinnamon (darchini)--Cinnamon is hot in the third degree. Its volatile oil is a great medicine for indigestion. It forms an ingredient in spice blends used as the basis of cooking in almost three-fourths of the world.

Citron (utrujj)--The Prophet (s.a.w.s.) is reported to have said, "The citron is like a true believer: good to taste and good to smell." Citron strengthens the heart, dispels sadness, removes freckles, satisfies hunger, and slows the flow of bile. The wife of the Prophet (s.a.w.s.) used to treat blind persons with citron dipped in honey. Citron is best taken about ten minutes after the conclusion of meals.

Cucumber (qitta')--Ripe cucumbers dispel heat and are diuretic. Eating dates with green cucumber is said to cause weight gain.

Cumin (kammun)--Cumin is very hot. It is reported to be the only spice or herb that travels through the stomach unaffected by digestion, until it reaches the liver. Cumin soaked in water, which is then drunk, is excellent for colic.

Dates, Dried (tamr)--The Prophet (s.a.w.s.) is reported to have said, "A house without dates has no food." Prophet Muhammad (s.a.w.s.) used to plant date trees himself. Dates should be eaten with almonds to annul any adverse effects. Fresh dates were the food eaten by Mary (r.a.), at the time of her delivery of the infant Jesus (a.s.). Said the Prophet (s.a.w.s.), "He who finds a date, let him break his fast on that. If he finds no date, let him break it on water. For verily that is purity."

Eggplant (badhinjan)--The dark variety of eggplant causes production of bile. Small amounts of it help piles. Eggplant's tendency to produce bile is corrected by eating it with meat dishes.

Eggs (baydah)--The best eggs are those of chickens, eaten soft, not hard-boiled. Egg white relieves pain of sunburn, aids healing of burns, and prevents scarring. Eggs are aphrodisiac.

Endive (hindiba')--The effects of endive change according to the season. Endive at the earliest time is best, and at the end of the growing season, virtually useless. The Hadith states: "Eat endives and do not belch, for verily there is not one day that drops of the water of Paradise do not fall upon them [endives]."

Fenugreek (hulbah)--It is reported the Prophet (s.a.w.s.) once said: "If my people knew what there is in fenugreek, they would have bought and paid its weight in gold." Fenugreek is hot and dry. As a tea it aids menstrual flow and is useful in colic and as a cleansing enema. Fenugreek strengthens the heart.

Fig (tin)--Fresh figs are preferred to dried. Although quite nourishing, they are very hot. The Prophet (s.a.w.s.) is reported to have said, "If you say that any fruit has come from Paradise, then you must mention the fig, for indeed it is the fruit of Paradise. So eat of it, for it is a cure for piles and helps gout."

Fish (samak)--Fresh-water fish are best, and those which feed on plant life, not mud and effluvia. Uncooked fish is hard to digest and produces imbalance of phlegm.

Garlic (thawm)--Garlic is hot in the third degree. It is used to dispel gas, promote menses, and expel afterbirth. It is excellent to correct cold intemperament, for dissolving phlegm, and the oil is used to treat insect bites. The eating of raw garlic and then visiting the mosque has been forbidden by the Prophet Muhammad (s.a.w.s.).

Ghee (clarified butter) (samn)--Ghee is the most fatty of all condiments. It is to be considered a medicinal additive to foods. Mixed with honey, ghee is said to be an antidote to poisons.

Ginger (zanjabil)--Ginger is mentioned in the Holy Qur'an (76:17). It is hot in the third degree, and is best for softening phlegm. It also aids digestion and strengthens sexual activity.

Henna (hinna)--One Hadith reports that nothing is dearer to Allah than henna. The Holy Prophet (s.a.w.s.) recommended it for many conditions: bruises, pain in the legs, infection of nails, burns, and to beautify the hair. Henna is noted for its great heat and its ability to excite the passions of love. The perfume made from henna flowers is considered to be one of the finest in the world. The dyeing of hands, nails, and feet is a common practice in the East, especially for weddings and feasts.

Honey ('asal)--Allah has said: "There comes forth, from within [the bee], a beverage of many colors in which there is a healing for you." Mixed with hot water, and taken in several small doses, honey is considered the best remedy for diarrhea. The Prophet (s.a.w.s.) once said, "By Him in whose hand is my soul, eat honey. For there is no house in which honey is kept for which the angels will not ask for mercy. If a person eats honey, a thousand remedies enter his stomach and a million diseases will come out. If a man dies and honey is found within him, fire will not touch his body [i.e., he will be immune from the burning of hell]." The Prophet (s.a.w.s.) himself used to drink a glass of honey and water each morning on an empty stomach. Honey is considered the food of foods, the drink of drinks, and the drug of drugs. It is used for creating appetite, strengthening the stomach, and eliminating phlegm; as a meat preservative, hair conditioner, eye salve, and mouthwash. The best honey is that produced in the spring; the second best is that of summer, and the least quality is produced in winter.

Lentils ('adas)--All lentils produce dryness. Small amounts should be eaten, as a side dish, for in quantity they are generally bad for the stomach. Hadith say that the eating of lentils produces a sympathetic heart, tears in the eyes, and removes pride.

Lettuce (khass)--Although cold, lettuce is considered the best nourishment of all vegetables. It softens a hard constitution and helps those who suffer delirium. It contradicts the sexual energy and dries up semen. Excess consumption of lettuce weakens the eyesight.

Marjoram, Sweet (marzanjush)--The Prophet (s.a.w.s.) is reported to have said that sweet marjoram is most excellent for anyone who has lost the sense of smell.

Meat (lahm)--Allah has said in the Qur'an (52:22): "And we will aid them with fruit and meat, such as they desire." The Prophet (s.a.w.s.) reportedly said that one who does not eat meat for forty consecutive days will waste away, whereas to eat meat for forty consecutive days will harden the heart. In other words, one should moderate the intake of meat. The most desirable of all meats is mutton, which is hot and moist in temperament. The best mutton is that of a male yearling; the best cut is a shoulder roast. Mutton should be cooked in some liquid, or it tends to dry out. Beef fat mixed with pepper and cinnamon acts as a tonic medicine. The meat of pigs is forbidden to eat. The consumption of horse flesh as a food is disputed. Avicenna said the flesh of camels, horses, and asses are the worst of all meats. Also prohibited for human consumption are beasts of prey, animals that possess canine teeth, and birds with hooked talons. Said the Prophet (s.a.w.s.): "Do not cut up meat with a knife upon the dish, for that is the way of non- Muslims. But grasp it in your fingers and so it will taste better." And, he said: "One sheep is a blessing; two sheep are two blessings; three sheep are wealth."

Melon (battikh)--Said the Prophet (s.a.w.s.): "Whenever you eat fruit, eat melon, because it is the fruit of Paradise and contains a thousand blessings and a thousand mercies. The eating of it cures every disease." Generally, the sweeter a melon, the greater its heat. Green varieties tend to be cold; the yellow, hot. The Prophet took melons with fresh dates. Melon purifies the bladder and the stomach, and improves the spinal fluid and eyesight. Melons should not be eaten first in a meal. Said the Prophet (s.a.w.s.): "None of your women who are pregnant and eat of watermelon will fail to produce offspring who are good in countenance and good in character."

Milk (laban)--Allah has mentioned milk to us, saying, "Rivers of milk the taste whereof does not change" (Qur'an 47:15). And again He said, "Pure milk, easy and agreeable to swallow for those who drink" (Qur'an 16:66). The Prophet Muhammad (s.a.w.s.) is said to have remarked that milk is irreplaceable and that he himself loved milk. Milk is composed of fat and water and milk solids (cheese). Together, these components are well suited to the constitution of humans. However, we should not take the milk of animals whose pregnancy lasts longer than that of humans. The milk of cows is best, for they feed off grasses. Said the Prophet (s.a.w.s.): "Drink milk, for it wipes away heat from the heart as the finger wipes away sweat from the brow. Furthermore, it strengthens the back, increases the brain, augments the intelligence, renews vision, and drives away forgetfulness." A milk diet is the best treatment there is for dropsy; however, anyone with fever must avoid milk.

Mint (nana)--The most subtle and refined of pot herbs, mint is heating and drying. Mint strengthens the stomach, cures hiccups, and encourages sexual activity. Placed in milk, mint will prevent it from turning to cheese.

Myrtle (as)--Cold in the second degree, myrtle is most used to stem diarrhea. Smelling the oil will cure headache caused by overheating. Myrtle tea with quince added is used for coughs.

Narcissus (narjis)--One Hadith says, "Smell a narcissus, even if only once a day or once a week or once a month or once a year or once a lifetime. For verily in the heart of man there is the seed of insanity, leprosy, and leukoderma. And the scent of narcissus drives them away."

Olives and Olive Oil (zayt and zaytun)--The older olive oil is, the hotter it becomes. Olive oil is an excellent treatment for the skin and hair, and it delays old age. Allah has said of the olive tree: "And a tree that grows out of Mount Sinai which produces oil and a condiment for those who eat. For olive oil is the supreme seasoning." Allah has also called it the Blessed

Tree (Qur'an 24:35). Green olives are the most nourishing, and counteract autointoxication. Black olives cause the spleen to overproduce bile and are hard on the stomach. Olive leaves can be chewed as treatment for inflammation of the stomach, skin ulcerations, and eruptions of herpes and hives.

Onion (basal)--Quite hot, the onion is a good corrective for all excess wetness. Onion improves the flavor of foods and eliminates phlegm. Raw onions cause forgetfulness. An excess of cooked onions causes headache and forgetfulness.

Parsley (karafs)--A Hadith states that eating parsley just before sleep will cause one to awaken with sweet breath and will eliminate or prevent toothache. Parsley stimulates sexual activity.

Peach (khu'kh)--Peaches generate cold, relax the stomach, and soften the bowels. A good laxative, peaches should be eaten before, rather than after, a meal.

Pistachio (fustaq)--It is said that to eat the heart of a pistachio nut with egg yolk will make the heart grow strong. The reddish skin stems diarrhea and vomiting.

Pomegranate (rumman)--Sweet pomegranates are preferred over the sour. The juice stems coughs. All kinds of pomegranates settle palpitations of the heart. Hazrat Ali (r.a.) said that the light of Allah is in the heart of whoever eats pomegranates. It is also reported that one who eats three pomegranates in the course of a year will be inoculated against ophthalmia for that year. Said the Prophet (s.a.w.s.): Pomegranate "cleanses you of Satan and from evil aspirations for forty days."

Quince (safarjal)--It is said that to eat quince on an empty stomach is good for the soul. Cold and dry, quince is astringent to the stomach, and it checks excessive menstrual flow. A few seeds placed in water will, after a few minutes, form a mucilage which is an excellent remedy for cough and sore throat, especially in the young. Quince is also excellent for pregnant women, gladdening their hearts. The Holy Prophet (s.a.w.s.) said: "Eat quince, for it sweetens the heart. For Allah has sent no prophet as His messenger without feeding him on the quince of Paradise. For quince increases the strength up to that of forty men."

Rhubarb (rawand)--Rhubarb is hot and dry, and best when picked fresh. It opens blockages of the liver and resolves chronic fever.

Rice (aruzz)--Next to wheat, rice is the most nourishing of whole grain foods. It is said eating rice increases pleasant dreams and the production of semen. Eating rice cooked in fat from sheep's liver is better and more effective than a major purging.

Saffron (zafaran)--Hot and dry, saffron is excellent for the blood and strengthening to the soul. It eases pains in the joints, but can cause great increase in the sex drive of young men.

Salt (milh)--Hot and dry in the third degree, salt, when taken moderately, is beautifying to the skin, giving it a soft glow. Salt causes vomiting when purging, and stimulates the appetite. Excessive use causes the skin to itch. The Prophet (s.a.w.s.) recommended beginning and ending each meal with a pinch of salt. He said: "From the one who begins a meal with salt, Allah wards off three hundred and thirty kinds of diseases, the least of which are lunacy, leprosy, bowel troubles, and toothache. The rest is pre-scribed in the supreme knowledge of Allah."

Senna (sana)--The best species of henna is that from the blessed city of Medina, where it grows plentifully. The chief property of senna is that it strengthens the heart without harshness. Its nobility has caused it to be referred to by the hakims as the Glory of Drugs. Its uses are many--in purgative infusions, decoctions, pills, enemas, and powders. Senna causes the bile to flow, and reaches to the very depths of the joints to balance the essences therein. The most effective use is as a tea, which can be made even more efficacious by adding violet blossoms and crushed red raisins. The Prophet (s.a.w.s.) recommended senna most highly, making a statement similar to the one about coriander: that it cures every disease except death itself.

Spinach (asfanakh)--Spinach is cold and moist, causing irritation to the chest and throat. Still, it softens the bowels. **Sugar (sukkar)**--Sugar is cold and moist. It is most often used in combination with other medicinal herbs, which carry the effects to the furthest point of an organ. Eating too much sugar creates disease of moisture.

Thyme (sa'tar)--In the time of the Prophet (s.a.w.s.), it was customary to fumigate houses by burning frankincense and thyme. Thyme is cold and dry in the third degree. An excellent digestive aid to heavy foods, thyme beautifies the complexion, annuls intestinal gas, and benefits coldness of the stomach and liver. When drunk as an infusion, it is said to kill tapeworms.

Vermicelli (itriyyah)--This food is hot and excessively moist, thus hard to digest. For those with very strong constitution, it provides excellent nourishment.

Vinegar (khall)--The Prophet Muhammad (s.a.w.s.) was reported to have once remarked that vinegar was the seasoning of all the prophets who came before him. Vinegar is both cold and hot, nearly balanced between the two. Mixed with rose water, it is an excellent remedy for toothache and headache. Vinegar dissolves phlegm. Another Hadith states that a house containing vinegar will never suffer from poverty.

Walnut (jawz)--Walnut is the hottest of nuts. Although hard to digest, when eaten with raisins it is the best remedy for winter cough. Avicenna said that walnuts cure the effects of poisons.

Water (ma')--The Prophet (s.a.w.s.) reportedly said: "The best drink in this world and the next is water." Water is moist and, because of this, slightly cooling. It extinguishes thirst and preserves the innate moisture of the body. It assists digestion of foods and absorption of nutrients. Said the Prophet (s.a.w.s.): "When you have a thirst, drink [water] by sips and do not gulp it down .... Gulping water produces sickness of the liver."

Wheat (hintah)--Wheat is somewhat hot, and balanced between dryness and moisture. The eating of raw wheat produces intestinal worms and gas. Wheat flour should be ground during the daytime. So praise be upon this Prophet who produced for us this marvelous knowledge which makes us see and understand and dazzles the wisest minds. Herein are proofs of Allah's kindness and benevolence upon His creatures, for He is the most kind and all-loving. May we serve Him with true vision. *Al-hamdu li-Lahi Rabb il-Alamin!* So all praise be to Allah, Lord of the Worlds! Amin!

Ref: http://www.deenislam.co.uk/

Allah's Food Pharmacy
"Allah is All-Knowing All-Wise"...Quran

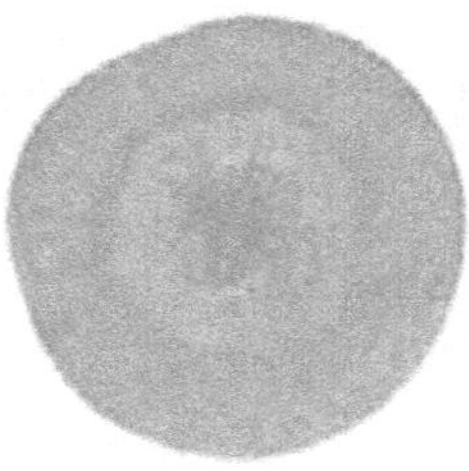

A sliced Carrot looks like the human eye The pupil, iris and radiating lines look just like the human eye...and YES science now shows that carrots greatly enhance blood flow to and function of the eyes.

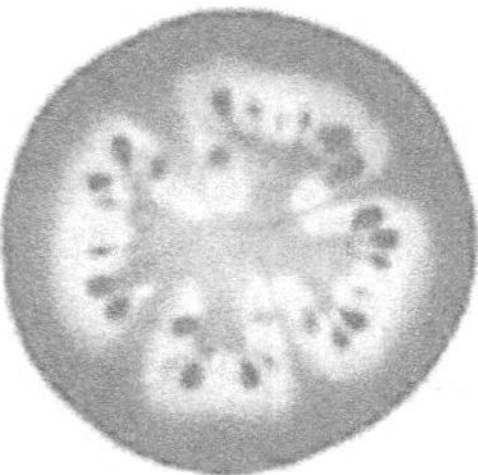

A Tomato has four chambers and is red. The heart is red and has four chambers. All of the research shows tomatoes are indeed pure heart and blood food.

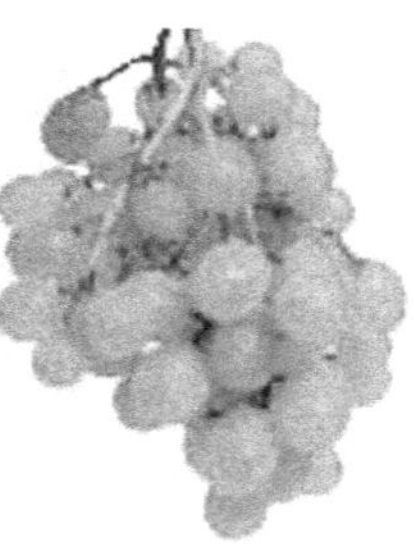

Grapes hang in a cluster that has the shape of the heart. Each grape looks like a blood cell and all of the research today shows that grapes are also profound heart and blood vitalizing food .

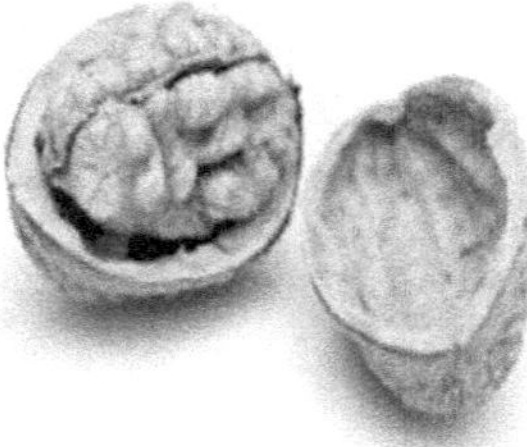

A Walnut looks like a little brain, a left and right hemisphere, upper cerebrums and lower cerebellums. Even the wrinkles or folds are on the nut just like the neo-cortex. We now know that walnuts help develop over 3 dozen neuron- transmitters for brain function.

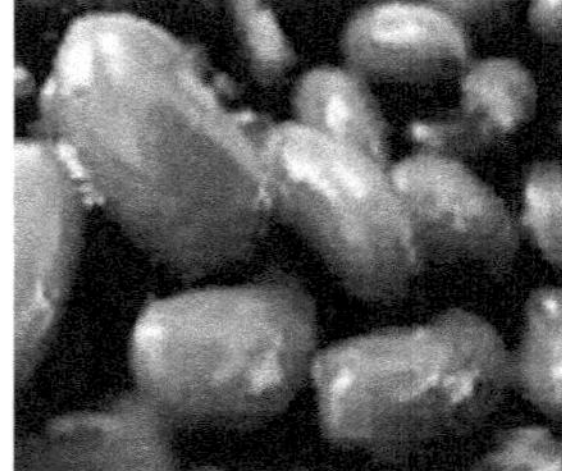

Kidney Beans actually heal and help maintain kidney function and yes, they look exactly like the human kidneys .

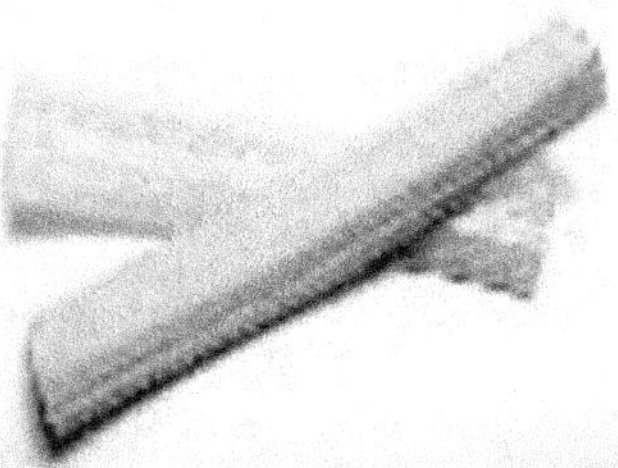

Celery, Bok Choy, Rhubarb and more look just like bones. These foods specifically target bone strength. Bones are 23% sodium and these foods are 23% sodium. If you don't have enough sodium in your diet the body pulls it from the bones, making them weak. These foods replenish the skeletal needs of the body.

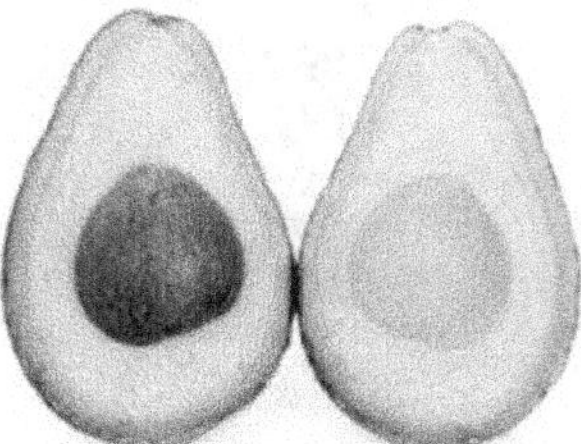

Eggplant, Avocadoes and Pears target the health and function of the womb and cervix of the female - they look just like these organs. Today's research shows that when a woman eats 1 avocado a week, it balances hormones, sheds unwanted birth weight and prevents cervical cancers. And how profound is this? .... It takes exactly 9 months to grow an avocado from blossom to ripened fruit. There are over 14,000 photolytic chemical constituents of nutrition in each one of these foods (modern science has only studied and named about 141 of them).

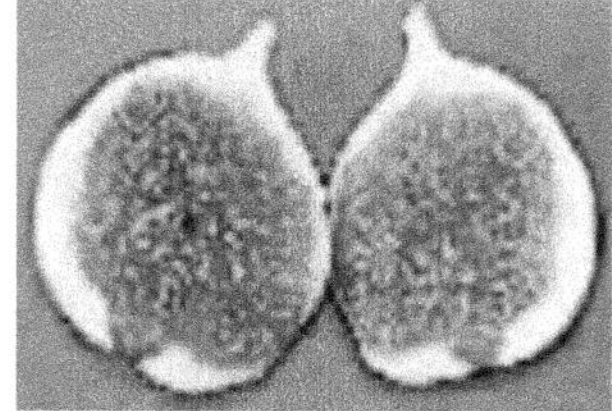

Figs are full of seeds and hang in twos when they grow. Figs increase the motility of male sperm and increase the numbers of Sperm cells to overcome male sterility.

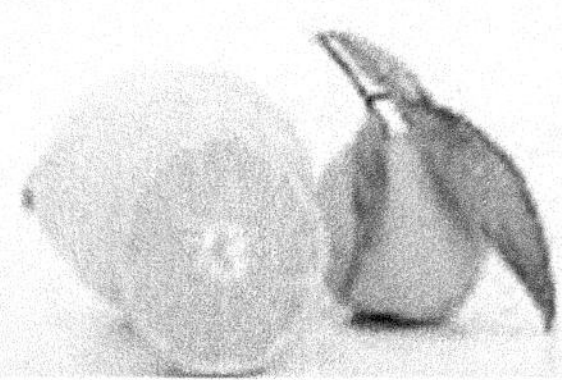

Grapefruits, Oranges, and other Citrus fruits look just like the mammary glands of the female and actually assist the health of the breasts and the movement of lymph in and out of the breasts.

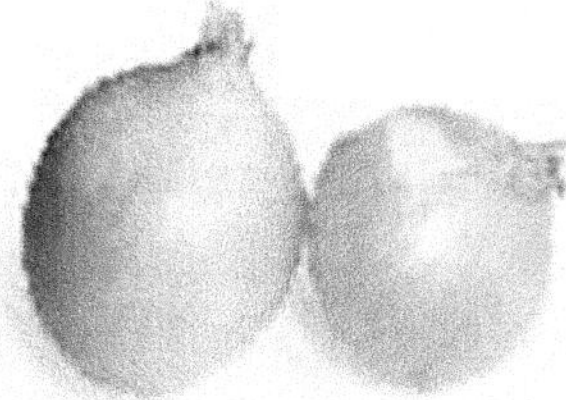

Onions look like body cells. Today's research shows that onions help clear waste materials from all of the body cells They even produce tears which wash the epithelial layers of the eyes.

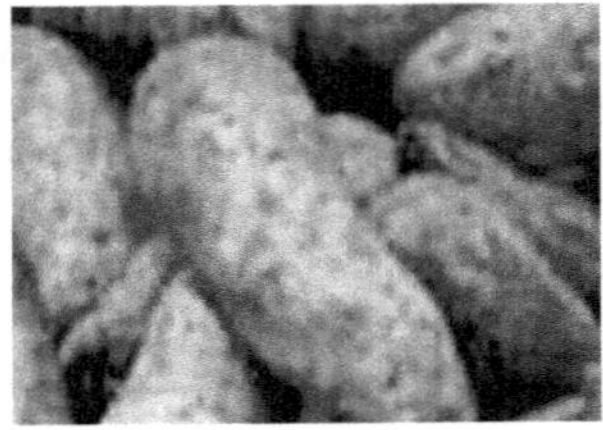

Sweet Potatoes look like the pancreas and actually balance the glycemic index of diabetics.

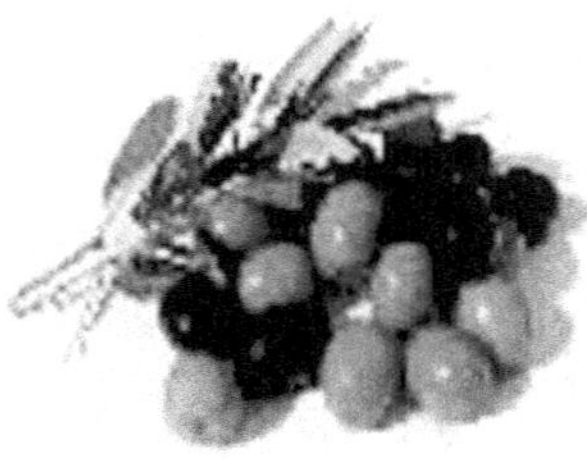

Olives assist the health and function of the ovaries

Then which of the favours of your Allah will ye deny? - [Quran 55:13]

Ref: http://www.islamcan.com/

9 Reasons to Drink a Cup of Honey Water

oney water is a remarkable drink, brimming with nutritional ingredients that will give your body energy and a health oost early in the morning. The best part is that all you need to make it is **a tablespoon of honey and a cup of kewarm water**. This delicious beverage is refreshing in the summer, a real treat in the winter and a true wonder cure fo variety of ailments. If you're still not convinced, here are 9 reasons you should make honey water your drink of choice in e morning.

Watch as Your Weight Drops

rinking honey water can help you lose weight, despite the sweetness of the drink. The natural sugar in the honey is much ealthier than the processed white sugar or corn syrup that is used in soft drinks, and is a healthier source of calories. By placing soft drinks with honey water you'll see a difference, although not overnight.

Maintain Healthy Bowels

ome people are shy about this topic, but there's no shame in discussing it. One cup of honey water a day will help your igestive system and keep you regular. The antibacterial properties of honey help prevent stomach aches and indigestion, nd help the body strengthen your stomach's lining.

Boost Your Immune System

oney is a natural antibacterial substance, and is also full of enzymes, vitamins and minerals — all of which help protect our body against germs, particularly organic honey. Several studieshave shown that Manuka honey, a unique honey made om a plant in New Zealand, can kill even antibiotic-resistant bacteria, and can be used as a natural cure for Helicobacter.

Reduce Allergy Symptoms

tudies have shown that eating locally-produced honey helps the body get accustomed to the local pollen, reducing lergy symptoms. If you suffer from seasonal allergies, drink a cup of water with local honey.

Healthy Energy Boost

ven mild dehydration can lead to you feeling tired, so imagine what a cup of water and honey can do to your energy vels. Unlike coffee, the energy boost doesn't subside. Instead, the body remains energized for a prolonged period of me.

Say Goodbye to Sore Throats

very grandmother will tell you that honey is the perfect remedy for a sore throat and coughing. Drinking honey water wi eate a type of coating around your esophagus, which will calm any coughing and pain, creating a smooth, pleasant nsation in your throat.

Detox

oney water helps flush toxins out of your body, both by helping your colon, as well as by its antibacterial properties. etoxing your body regularly helps you feel better and prevents infections. To boost the detox, add some freshly squeeze mon to your honey water. Lemons too contain antibacterial properties, are diuretic, and aid liver functions.

Less Bloating

eeling bloated and gassy? A cup of honey water will help neutralize the gas, reducing the bloated sensation. It's highly commended that you drink it after a big meal.

Keeps Your Heart Healthy

bove all of its other advantages, honey water helps in raising your "good" cholesterol (HDL) levels. Furthermore, it revents the body from producing stress hormones, which put pressure on the heart and cardiovascular system.

5 Foods That'll Help You Sleep

Lack of sleep can ruin a lot of things: our mood, our patience, our focus and our sense of enjoyment in life. We've all had those sleepless nights. But taking sleeping pills is usually a problematic strategy, because they don't give you the same natural sleep that strengthens you, and they can become quite addictive too. Better to eat something that will help you fall into a relaxing, renewing, deep sleep.

Here are five recommended foods to put you to sleep:

Frozen Bananas

Frozen bananas can be turned into a thick and tasty ice-cream. All you need is the right technique of consistent mixing. The idea is to mix for several minutes until the bananas turn into a creamy delight. Add a handful of chopped peanuts for an extra tryptophan boost (a chemical that is known to relieve tension and put you to sleep) and you have a great combination. Not only will the potassium in the bananas help you fall asleep faster, it can also prevent you waking up for no reason in the middle of the night.

Low Fat Popcorn

The carbs in popcorn will help your body better utilize tryptophan. This happens because the tryptophan is converted into serotonin, which is responsible for putting you to sleep and waking you up every day. Since a heavy meal about 2 hours before sleep can actually keep you awake at times, a low-calorie popcorn bowl is a recommended treat for late night snacks. If you want to add some flavor, we suggest some curry powder or garlic, instead of butter.

Halibut

The halibut fish comes with two great sleeping aids: tryptophan and vitamin B6. It has a meaty, gentle texture - recommended for sea food lovers.

Other foods rich in Tryptophan:

Chicken, Beef, soy, yogurt, bananas, peanuts and eggs.

Mango shake

Mangos are packed with antioxidants, proteins, and vitamins and are also a natural sweet that can help banish your sugar cravings.

To make a mango shake:

Cut up a fresh mango and put it in the blender. Add a scoop-full of ice, a small scoop of low-fat Greek yogurt and just a little splash of milk or water. To make it a little sweeter, you can add a bit of honey. And if you don't like mangoes, the same can be done with strawberries in the winter and watermelons in the summer.

Dried Cherries

A handful of dried cherries won't just provide you with a dose of carbs and serotonin, it is also one of the better-known sources of melatonin - a sleep-inducing hormone (also essential in preventing jet-lag). If that's not enough for you, dried cherries are also packed with antioxidants.

Ref: http://www.ba-bamail.com/

10 Super Foods That Prevent Memory Loss

The older you get, the more important it is to take care of your brain in order for it to function properly. The human brain relies on a steady supply of nutrients from our diet, blood sugar and oxygen, all vital components for preventing such mental disorders as Alzheimer's and dementia.

The brain is responsible for controlling all movement, thought processing and the sensations in the human body. It is a gigantic memory-storing warehouse, capable of holding over 2.5 petabytes of data, which is approximately three million hours of your favorite T.V shows and movies.

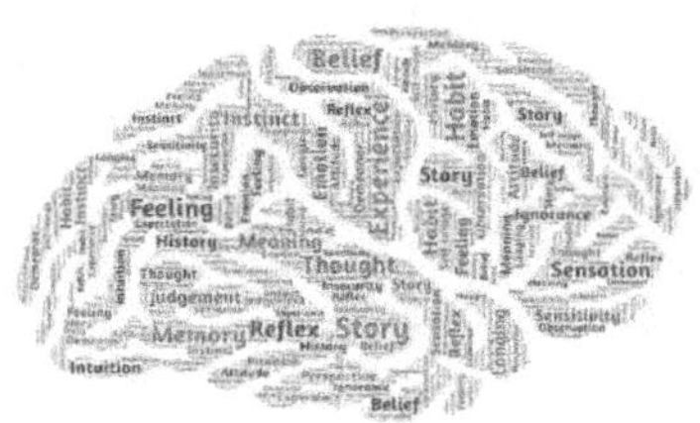

The brain regulates every single movement your body makes, from raising your arms in the air to walking in a straight line and blinking your eyes. So take care of it, learn about 10 super foods that can help fight off mental illnesses, increase memory power and keep your brain healthier.

10 Super Foods That Help Boost Brain Power

1. **Dark Chocolate -** Chocolate lovers will be pleased to know that this delicious treat can also be used to increase memory power and even lower cholesterol. Dark chocolate contains many anti-aging and anti- inflammatory properties, which help increase proper blood flow. Enjoy a piece of dark chocolate after dinner and look for the versions at the supermarket that contain 70% cocoa.

2. **Blueberries -** Blueberries are a delicious memory enhancing snack, boosting many cognitive functions. Blueberries contain high levels of flavonoids, which are vital components that keep the brain protected from Parkinson's disease and dementia. You can mix a handful of blueberries together with your yogurt, or eat a half cup of them daily.

3. **Walnuts -** Walnuts are known to improve memory and thinking abilities since they contain very high levels of omega-3 fatty acids. Omega-3 fatty acids play a critical role in the proper functioning of neurotransmitters, keeping your mind super sharp. They provide essential nutrients and keep the oxygen properly flowing throughout blood vessels in the brain. Add 1/2 cup of chopped walnuts to homemade fruit salads, oatmeal or simply eat a handful of them raw.

4. **Wild Salmon -** Salmon is one of the healthiest super foods you can eat. It is a rich source of omega-3 fatty acids, many essential vitamins and DHA (docosahexaenoic acid), which can significantly reduce the risk for Alzheimer's disease. Choose wild salmon as opposed to the farmed version, since it contains fewer levels of mercury and PCB contamination.

5. **Turmeric -** The dark yellow turmeric spice contains high levels of the curcumin property, which can prevent Alzheimer's disease and other serious illnesses from forming in the body. It is used as a natural healing treatment for toothaches, various stomach disorders and clogged arteries. Turmeric also improves cognitive functions, such as problem-solving and reasoning.

6. **Spinach -** Spinach is loaded with all the essential vitamins your brain requires to function properly. It contains high amounts of potassium, which helps to promote the electrical conductivity going on in the brain. Spinach also protects against fatigue, drowsiness and even dementia. Make sure you include this incredible leafy green vegetable to your diet.

7. **Tomatoes -** Tomatoes help destroy free radical damage to cells, which can lead to severe mental disorders and even cancer. Tomatoes protect against memory loss since they contain high amounts of the lycopene antioxidant property. There are many ways to enjoy this robust vegetable. You can add them to your salad, prepare a homemade tomato sauce or use them in a healthy low-fat soup dish.

8. **Broccoli** - Broccoli contains a memory boosting compound known as choline, which can increase the growth of new brain cells and neural connections. Broccoli also reduces bad cholesterol levels, improves bone density and protects from cancer. They are also great sources of vitamin C and keep you protected from the common cold. Eat a cupful of broccoli at least three times per week to reap their incredible health benefits.

9. **Acorn Squash** - Winter squash is a rich source of folic acid, which allows for quick transmission of information through nerve cells. Squash contains high levels of the B-12 vitamin that protects against nerve damage. You won't be forgetting important details any time soon with a helping of winter squash. They can be baked, roasted or pureed as well.

10. **Green Tea** - Green tea contains plenty of immune-strengthening antioxidants, which help you concentrate better and stay healthy overall. Drink 2-3 cups of green tea each day to prevent memory loss and protect against mental diseases. You can increase these health benefits by adding a squirt of freshly squeezed lemon juice, a few ginger roots and a dash of honey to it.

H/T: top10homeremedies.com

The Health Benefits of Eating a Mediterranean Diet

The Mediterranean diet is supposed to be the healthiest in the world, and that was reason enough for me to switch to it!
The diet has been scientifically proven by numerous studies to promote good health in those who eat it, lowering the risk of developing chronic and potentially fatal diseases.
Furthermore, the diet has also been shown to extend a healthy lifespan in aging adults. This is because the calorie intake from a Mediterranean diet is lower than other diets, and helps to preserve memory in addition to lowering serious illness risk.
A Swiss study in particular compared participants over the age of 70 who adhere to a Mediterranean diet with those who ate more meat and animal products. It showed that those who ate a Mediterranean diet were found to have a 20% higher chance of living longer.
In practice, study participants that ate a Mediterranean diet were shown to live two to three years longer on average than those who did not.

What it Consists Of

Lots of fresh fruit and vegetables are staples of the Mediterranean diet, as are legumes, nuts and whole grains. Herbs and spices are primarily used in order to flavor food. While olive oil is one of the main sources of fat in this diet. Eggs, fish, poultry and red meat are also eaten in small amounts.

Other Mediterranean Diet Benefits

Following a Mediterranean diet is purported to reduce the risk of Alzheimer's disease, cancer, heart disease, high cholesterol, high triglycerides and Parkinson's disease. This is because of the healthy unsaturated fat intake from consuming nuts and olive oil as part of the diet. Further contributing to lowering these risks are the high fiber and nutrient content contained in the fruits and vegetables that make up a significant part of it.

How to Make Your Diet More Mediterranean

1. **Cook at home more often**
   Stock up on whole, unprocessed ingredients so you can control portion sizes, salt and calories. Stock your pantry and freezer with Mediterranean-inspired staples such as canned tomatoes, whole-wheat pasta and frozen vegetables.

2. **Get your protein from beans and fish**
   This doesn't mean you have to stop eating meat completely — swap some of it out for beans, nuts and other plants. This will help you lower your saturated fat intake while adding healthy nutrients, such as flavonols, to your intake. Start by aiming to make a plant-based dinner once or twice each week. Alternatively, try and make whole grains or vegetables the focus of a meal, only using meat as flavoring.

3. **Feel the love for olive oil**
   You should give heart-healthy olive oil precedence over butter or lard. When it comes to vegetables, you can drizzle them in olive oil to bring out their natural flavor. Olive oils that are yellow or Green in color and have a pronounced odor and taste are the ones to go for.

4. **Allow yourself a glass of wine**
   If you enjoy a glass of wine, try and incorporate it into your meal and avoid drinking the rest of the time. Drinking wine in moderation increases good cholesterol, regulates blood sugar and even helps with digestion. Red wine in particular will also give you a healthy dose of resveratrol, which is good for the heart.

Content Sources: <u>Natural News</u>, <u>LiveStrong</u>, <u>eatingwell.com</u>

The Mind Diet: Eating for a Healthy Brain

Diet and nutrition may play an influential part when it comes to the health of your brain. New research suggests what you eat can affect your thinking skills and slow down or speed up the onset of dementia and Alzheimer's. Researchers believe that nutrition can play a role in preventing the brain from shrinking as people age. Recent studies observed that older adults who followed a Mediterranean diet showed higher brain volume than their peers who followed other diets.

The **Mind diet**, developed by Martha C Morris at the Rush Medical Center in Chicago, is a combination of the Mediterranean diet and the DASH diet (Dietary Approaches to Stop Hypertension). This progressive diet merges the healthy practices of both eating plans to help benefit the brain.

This new super-diet recommends plenty of fruits, vegetables, nuts, and legumes. It advises whole grains over refined ones, moderate amounts of wine (a glass or two per day) and emphasizes fish, poultry and seeds. The diet discourages saturated fats, added sugars and salt. There is little dairy, eggs and red meat, but it includes plenty of olive oil.

This eating style can reduce inflammation and plaque buildup in the brain. Inflammation has been linked to Alzheimer's and other chronic diseases. A typical Western diet lacks diversity and is high in sugar, salt, saturated fats and processed food, which all lead to inflammation. The nutrients in this diet may block pathways to Alzheimer's. Foods such as olive oil, grapes, berries, plums, apricots, leafy green vegetables and walnuts have been observed to reduce plaque buildup in the brain.

The Mind diet also favors anti-inflammatory foods and cuts out inflammatory foods. For example, omega-3 fatty acids found in fish, seeds, nuts, and olive oil are anti-inflammatory. A study of 1,200 adults over the age of 65, who closely followed a Mediterranean diet for 4 years, were observed to have lowered their risk of developing Alzheimer's by 34%, compared to their peers.

Alzheimer's has also been called "type 3 diabetes" by some researchers. Diets high in sugar increase the risk of developing diabetes, which in turn increases the risk for Alzheimer's. Insulin resistance caused by type 2 diabetes results in tissue damage, mental decline and other early signs of Alzheimer's. The Mind diet recommends cutting out added sugars altogether.

An additional contributor to developing Alzheimer's is oxidative stress. This is when the immune system can't stop the damaging effects of toxins that enter or develop in the body. There is evidence that diets rich in antioxidant foods combat oxidative stress. The Mind diet recommends foods like blueberries and spinach, which are rich in antioxidants.

The Mind diet also advocates herbs and spices, another source of lowering inflammation and oxidative stress. Research suggests that cinnamon reduces brain plaque while a daily dose of 30g saffron is as effective at fighting Alzheimer's symptoms as the prescription drug donepezil. Turmeric was also found to be good at combating inflammation and oxidative stress.

Researchers are exploring whether the results of specific diets, like the Mind diet, are caused by a single food or nutrient or a combination of several foods and nutrients. Scientists are looking at all healthy habits that prevent a decline in thinking skills, such as the long-term effect of exercise on brain function. Many researchers believe the prevention of cognitive decline includes a combination of diet, mental and physical exercise, sleep, and social engagement.

Ref: H/T: www.webmd.com

Herbs & Spices that Lower Blood Pressure

Taking care of our health can be hard work at times, even if it's just taking prescription medication since they can come with some very unpleasant side effects. If you're suffering from high blood pressure, you'll be happy to learn that regular consumption of certain spices can lower your blood pressure without pesky side effects (other than deliciousness!). You're going to want to add these spices to your daily meals to enjoy their fantastic properties.

Garlic

A popular ingredient in many dishes, Garlic is also one of the best plants for treating high blood pressure. It naturally lowers blood pressure and is also beneficial for keeping a healthy heart, so don't be afraid to add it to your food.

Hawthorn

This plant is rich in flavonoids that help restore the cardiovascular system. Hawthorn has been used to lower blood pressure for a very long time, and various studies have found that it is highly effective when taken with medicine. It can be taken as a supplement or as an infusion.

Linden / Lime Blossoms

Linden (Lime in the UK) blossoms are a supplement made out of dried Tilia tree flowers. These flowers' benefits include relief of common cold symptoms, stomach aches, and lowering high blood pressure. To effectively lower your blood pressure, drink 1-2 cups of linden blossom infusion on a daily basis.

Saffron

Although Saffron is a rare and expensive spice, it's an excellent choice for lowering blood pressure. Studies have found that regular consumption of saffron helps normalize blood pressure significantly.

Ginger

Ginger is a popular ingredient in many dishes around the world, and studies have found it to be very effective in lowering high blood pressure. For the best results, add fresh ginger to your food, or as an infusion.

Cayenne Pepper

The common ingredient in hot peppers is capsaicin, and aside from making food hot, it is also effective at long-term lowering of the blood pressure, so you don't have to have it every day. Unless you love the spiciness, consider adding it to your dishes once or twice a week.

Ginkgo Biloba

This herb grows on the mountains of China and has been used there to improve blood circulation for many generations. What ginkgo does is expand the arterial walls, which has also been shown to aid in improving memory and alertness.

Turmeric

This yellow spice is known as a powerful anti-inflammatory, is effective at lowering cholesterol levels, and reduces the likeliness of blood clots. It has been found to be very effective in lowering blood pressure, particularly in people who suffer from autoimmune diseases. Don't be shy, add this terrific herb to your dishes regularly.

Valerian

Valerian grows year-round across Europe and Asia. It is known for its ability to relax the muscles that surround the blood vessels, which improves blood circulation throughout the body. Valerian is usually available as a supplement or in root form for infusions. Please note that it is NOT recommended for pregnant or breastfeeding women.

Yarrow

This European plant is internationally known for its muscle-relaxing and spasm-relieving properties. It causes the body to sweat and is considered to be effective in reducing blood pressure.

Olive Leaves

The leaves of the olive tree can be used both fresh and dried (for an infusion or as an essential oil), to strengthen and bolster the heart and blood vessels. The active ingredient in the leaves is oleuropein – an elenolic acid that protects the heart. Additionally, the leaves contain flavonoids, which keep the old ticker working regularly by expanding your blood vessels.

These natural herbs and roots are a great natural treatment for lowering your blood pressure, but before using them as an alternative, please consult with your family doctor first. Additionally, there are a few other plants that can help with your blood pressure:

Terminalia Arjuna – Helps to regulate heart rate and blood pressure.

Scutellaria – Used in traditional Chinese medicine to ease chi-blocks to the heart.

Cinnamon – A daily consumption of 1-2 grams of cinnamon can lower high blood pressure in diabetics.

Hydrocotyle Asiatica – A common plant around the world, it is also known to improve the blood cycle and strengthens the heart muscles. Can be used both fresh and dried.

Lavender – A strong disinfectant with other benefits, such as invigorating and strengthening your body, as well as improvement of blood circulation.

Nutmeg – Used in traditional Chinese medicine to improve blood circulation.

For a complete treatment, combine more vegetables and other foods rich in minerals and vitamins in your diet. Put an emphasis on Q10 coenzyme, vitamins B6, B12, C, and E. This will help you maintain a healthy blood pressure.

The information in this article is not a substitute for medical treatment. If you wish to change your medicinal care, consult with your physician first.

Ref: http://www.ba-bamail.com/

The Secret Remedies of Different Cultures

Sri Lanka

Coconut to battle fat

A resident of Sri Lanka eats, on average, about 116 coconuts a year, and the people living in this tropical paradise have the lowest risk of obesity in the world.

The reason? Coconut oil is rich in fatty acids of medium length that absorb swiftly in the body, accelerate the rate of metabolism and calorie burn in the body, and give a lasting sense of being full. A study conducted on the topic found that consuming about 2 spoons of coconut oil a day, 170 gram or 300ml, can help the person lose about 1.3 kg a month.

Austria

Yoga to beat insomnia

The use of yoga to decrease stress is known, but in Austria it is also used to battle insomnia. According to a study by Pennsylvania University, a yoga exercise of about 20 minutes a day is just as useful as taking a sleeping pill. In addition, the yoga reduces stress, chronic tension and depressed moods within two weeks time. The reason is that the gentle stretching and controlled breathing make the body secrete the GABA neurotransmitter, which has a calming effect on the nervous system.

Indonesia

Ginger to boost cardio health

Indonesia has the highest consumption rate of ginger in the world. Locals don't just throw this tasty root into their foods, the use it to make tea, candy, bread and other foodstuffs. They see it as a plant with great benefits for the heart - and are now backed up by science. Researchers from Stanford claim that half a tablespoon of ginger a day will reduce risk of clogged arteries by 27%, and it is also twice as efficient as aspirin at preventing dangerous blood clots.

India

Turmeric to stabilize blood sugar levels

In India, the turmeric is not only a tasty spice, but a medicinal material used to treat high blood sugar levels. Studies have shown that the active ingredient in turmeric - curcumin - reduces and stabilizes the levels of sugar in the blood, as well as helps the pancreas secrete insulin when the blood sugar levels rise. One must take at least half a teaspoon a day for results.

Japan

Mushrooms to control cholesterol levels

Edible mushrooms are considered food in Japan, but even more so as medicine. The average Japanese woman consumes about 8 kilograms (17 pounds) of mushrooms a year. Adding mushrooms to your daily diet can help reduce the levels of cholesterol by up to 30%, according to a study by Pennsylvania University.

England

Mustard to battle muscle pain

Soaking in a hot bath with mustard seeds is a traditional English remedy for muscle pain. The unique build of the mustard causes the body to secrete toxins through the skin pores, improve blood flow, relax tense muscles and help heal damaged tissue

Germany

Chamomile tea to battle gas

This is an old German remedy that now has science backing it up. Stanford University researchers found that sipping 2 glasses of chamomile tea a day can reduce that bloated feeling as well actual gasses in the digestion system. The chamomile reduces the secretion of cortisol, a hormone secreted during times of stress and causes stomach cramps.

Russia

Garlic vs. Viral infections

Russians use garlic when they need to battle colds, the flu and most other infectious diseases. A study conducted by the University of Florida recommends consuming one clove of garlic a day. According to the study, garlic contains organic composites that help fight viral infections, and consuming one clove of garlic a day can decrease the risk of infection by 43%.

Finland

Coffee to battle depression

The Finnish are among the biggest coffee consumers in the world - each of them sips, on average, 1,640 cups of coffee a year (that's more than 4 cups a day). When coffee first arrived in Finland in the 18th century, it was sold as anti- depression medicine.

Drinking 2 cups of coffee a day can reduce depressed moods by 34%, drinking 3 - by 42%. According to the study, the combination of caffeine with the antioxidants found in coffee, energizes the brain and causes it to secrete anti- depression hormones such as serotonin and dopamine.

New Zealand

Honey to battle sinus and throat infections.

Unpasteurized honey is a very common remedy in New Zealand for taking care of inflammation in the sinuses and throat. According to researchers from the universities of Illinois and Amsterdam, the natural antibiotics and the

enzymes in the unpasteurized honey destroy almost 100% of germs and viruses - including those that cause throat ache and sinus inflammations.

Egypt

Coriander vs. food poisoning

Coriander is one of the oldest spices in the world, and a traditional Egyptian medicine for stomach problems. Now, a study published in the farming and food chemistry journal shows that the seeds of the coriander hasten the healing process after suffering from inflammation of the bowels and other stomach problems.

Coriander kills the bacteria responsible for stomach pain, including E-Coli and Salmonellae, by creating holes in the outer shell. So next time you have a really upset stomach, mix one spoon of coriander powder in hot water and soak for 5 minutes. Drink 3 glasses of this a day until you feel better.

Ref: http://www.ba-bamail.com/

The Health Benefits of Guava

Guavas are found in the tropics, and invoke images of vacations, summer parties and island life, but this tasty fruit is more than a celebratory food. *This* fruit is bursting with healthy vitamins and minerals and can be used to treat many serious ailments. You can recognize guavas by their yellow, green or maroon skins and creamy white or pink pulp.

1. **Weight loss and gain**
   Guava is a winning fruit for its many great benefits. If you're trying to lose weight, guavas are not a fruit you need to give up. In fact, this snack-sized fruit can satisfy your appetite while adding few calories, low amounts of carbohydrates and no cholesterol to your diet. Also, compared to other fruit, it adds a low dose of sugar. Guavas also offer a great source of vitamins, proteins, roughage, fibers and minerals. For lean people trying to gain weight, this fruit is also beneficial as it promotes the healthy absorption of nutrients and its substantial nutrients regulate one's metabolism.

2. **Blood pressure and Diabetes**
   Guavas are hypoglycemic and rich in fiber, which help reduce blood pressure. Dietary fibers maintain the blood's fluidity and prevent it from thickening, which can worsen blood pressure. Foods lacking in fiber (for example refined flour) increase blood pressure because they convert to sugar more quickly. This can help fight or even prevent diabetes. The fiber regulates the sugar being absorbed by the body and the risk of both high spikes and drops in the body's insulin and glucose levels is reduced.

3. **Diarrhea, dysentery, and gastroenteritis**
   The abundant astringent (substances that contract body tissue) makeup of raw guava and guava leaves helps loosen the bowels and reduce the symptoms of diarrhea and gastroenteritis. Being highly alkaline, the guavas act as a disinfectant, removing excess mucus from the intestines and inhibiting microbial growth. For these reasons, guavas can also be used to treat dysentery. The guavas' plentiful supply of vitamin C, carotenoids and potassium can also boost your digestive system.

4. **Thyroid health**
   A good substance for regulating the thyroid's metabolism is copper, which guavas have plenty of. The thyroid glands regulate important hormones and organ system functions, which helps maintain a healthy balance in your body.

5. **Healthy brains**
   Also present in guavas are high amounts of vitamins B3 and B6. These both have benefits for the health of your brain. B3, which is also called niacin, is known to help increase blood flow and stimulate cognitive function, while B6 helps preserve normal nerve function.

6. **Scurvy**
   Guava is your best source for vitamin C. In fact, it has four times the amount of Vitamin C found in oranges, which are regarded as the go-to food for this vitamin. The concentration of vitamin C can prevent scurvy, a disease caused by a deficiency of this vitamin.

7. **Constipation**
   The seeds of guavas, either ingested whole or chewed, are excellent laxatives. In addition to the fruits' substantial amount of dietary fiber, guavas are advantageous for treating constipation. These two sources cleanse your intestines and excretory system and help your body retain water, helping you achieve healthy bowel movements. Frequently snacking on guavas, then, can be beneficial for proper digestion.

8. **Colds and coughs**
   Drinking the juice of guavas and fresh guava fruit helps in fighting colds and coughs. The astringent quality can lessen mucus, disinfect the respiratory tract, throat, and lungs and reduce microbial activity. The substantial amounts of iron and vitamin C in guavas also help treat viral infections. It's advised to avoid eating overly ripe guavas when you have a cold or cough, as they can actually aggravate them.

9. **Eyesight**

The considerable quantities of vitamin A in guavas are extremely beneficial for the health of your vision. This helps slow down macular degeneration, the growth of cataracts and can even improve one's eyesight deterioration once it has begun.

10. **Cancer prevention**

Guava is also valuable in your diet as a preventative measure against cancerous growths and metastasis. The high levels of an antioxidant called lycopene has been shown to reduce the risk of prostate cancer and inhibit the growth of breast cancer cells. Guava leaf oil is another anti- proliferative extract from the guava plant that has proven effective in reducing cancer growth

11. **Skincare**

Guavas are also fantastic at improving skin texture and keeping your skin looking fresh. Guavas are full of astringents, particularly in fresh fruit and the leaves of the plant. If you rinse your skin with a guava decoction, the fruit can tone and tighten areas of loose skin. Eating the fruit also provides a rich source of vitamins A, B, C, as well as potassium, which are excellent antioxidants and detoxifiers. They can keep your skin glowing, prevent premature aging and wrinkles, and can speed up the healing process of wounds.

Ref: H/T: www.organicfacts.net

8 Very Healthy and Very Tasty Tropical Fruit!

We're used to hearing that tasty and healthy rarely go together, but these tropical fruit easily prove otherwise. In rain forests and tropical climates around the world grow treasures rich in both nutrients and taste - **meet 8 easy to come by exotic fruit that really pack a healthy punch!** Remember: Consume these fruit in their raw form, not as dried fruit (high in sugar) or as canned.

Asai

This fruit comes to us straight from the Amazonas area and was brought to the rest of the world by hikers from other countries. The asai is a type of palm tree with a small purple fruit that is considered a 'antioxidant bomb'. The extremely high level of antioxidants the asai contains have made it a very sought after anti-aging tool, in addition to its exotic taste. Additionally, the asai is a fruit that is rich in protein and contains Omega 6 and Omega 9 fatty acids. Due to its low sugar content, it is also safe for diabetes patients to eat.

Guava The guava mainly grows in the Caribbeans and the nations of South and Central America. In addition to vitamins, potassium and fiber, the guava is also a rich source of potassium, an element needed for a variety of biological processes in the body. The guava contains anti-bacterial materials as well as substances that lower the blood sugar levels. It is also known to relax clenched muscles and aids the digestive system.

Mango

The mango may not be so exotic in all places, but it originally comes from the rain forests of India and China. Like other tropical fruit, the mango is rich in vitamins A and C, potassium and fiber, as well as antioxidants. The mango fruit also contains a lot of iron, crucial for burning energy and every action the body takes. Almost every part of the mango tree can be used for medicinal purposes.

Carambola

This wax-textured, star shaped fruit is not very common, but can still be found in specialized fruit shops. It comes from the tropical climates of South East Asia. Each fruit is about 40 calories and is a great source of vitamin C essential for the immune system, especially during the winter, as well as a fantastic source of vitamin A, which is known to improve sight and skin function.

Kiwi

The hairy fruit with the sweet & sour taste comes from South China. The kiwi is among the fruit with the highest Vitamin C content in the world, twice more than oranges. It is a great source of magnesium, essential for the heart and blood systems, and also a fat-free source of vitamin E, which is rare in fruit. It is also known as a great natural remedy for the flu and the various parts of the plant (including the fruit), aid in the battle against joint pain, kidney stones and various types of cancer.

Papaya

From Central America comes this beautiful orange fruit, packed full of great nutrients. It has a unique enzyme called papain which helps to disassemble protein and helps in renewing tissue. In traditional Chinese medicine, the papaya is a remedy for constipation. It also contains a lot of folic acid, which helps keep our DNA, bone marrow and blood cells intact.

Passionfruit (aka passiflora)

This fruit has become more popular in recent years, and some even grow it in their back yard for its vitamin A and C content , for its potassium levels and its fiber. It is only about 16 calories a fruit and is known to have great relaxation effects, and so we recommend eating it before sleep to treat insomnia. It is also chock full of antioxidants.

Pineapple

Like many of the others on this list, the pineapple originally comes from the tropical areas of South America - mainly Brazil, Bolivia and Paraguay. The pineapple also contains a lot of vitamin A and C, but what's special about it is the bromelain - an enzyme that has strong anti-bacterial properties and is essential to the digestive system. It is even used in mainstream medicine, but is best taken directly from raw food.

http://www.ba-bamail.com/

Dark Chocolate: Nature's Delicious Medicine

Finally some good news about your favorite treat. A lot of research has gone into chocolate consumption and it turns out its really good for your health. It seems daily doses of dark chocolate can keep the doctor far away.

Don't go stuffing your face just yet. While dark chocolate has an abundance of benefits experts warn that it also highly fattening and can often be filled with lots of added sugars. Nonetheless, the delicious food has many advantages, you'd be crazy not to want to eat it.

1. **Rich in nutrients**
    Dark chocolate is rich in many of the vitamins and minerals that are vital for your body's functioning. It has high concentrations of magnesium, iron, potassium, and copper. Magnesium helps prevent high blood pressure, type 2 diabetes and other heart disease while iron protects against anemia. Both potassium and copper prevent stroke and cardiovascular disease. Dark chocolate, with at least 70% cocoa, contains a fair amount of fiber, manganese, phosphorus, zinc and selenium, all daily required minerals from your diet.

2. **mproves blood circulation and blood pressure**
    A significant benefit of dark chocolate is that it's good for your heart and blood because it may improve your blood flow and lower blood pressure. Dark chocolate contains chemical compounds called flavanols. These stimulate the lining of arteries to produce a gas called nitric oxide. This gas sends signals to the blood vessels to relax, which lowers resistance to blood flow and in turn this helps reduce blood pressure. Lower blood flow reduces your chance of blood clots from forming and prevents arteriosclerosis, the hardening of arteries.

3. **It's good for insulin resistance**
    Another benefit of dark chocolate is that it's a good option for those with diabetes as it has a low glycemic index, so eating it doesn't make your blood sugar levels rise. Dark chocolate has flavonoids, plant pigments, which are usually removed from chocolate because of their bitter taste. They help your cells function normally and retrain your body to use insulin effectively, reducing insulin resistance.

4. **It can reduce cholesterol**
    Researchers have found that regularly eating dark chocolate lowers the LDL cholesterol. This is the "bad" cholesterol which is dangerous when oxidized. It can inflame your arteries, and promote heart attack or stroke risk. Dark chocolate contains powerful antioxidants which protect against oxidative damage. Dark chocolate has also been shown to increase HDL, the "good" cholesterol.

5. **It improves the health of your skin**
    Dark chocolate can also be good for your skin's health. Flavonoids in dark chocolate increase skin density and hydration, and improve your blood flow to your skin. Flavonoids offer some protection against sun-induced damage and can thwart off the reddening effect of burns, however, they can't replace a good layer of sunscreen.

6. **Protection for your teeth**
    Dark chocolate contains Theobromine, which eliminates bacteria and hardens tooth enamel. If you practice good dental hygiene, dark chocolate can actually lower your risk of getting cavities.

7. **It can treat coughs**
    Theobromine is also a mild stimulant and does wonders for suppressing coughs. This chemical compound blocks the sensory nerves from activity and this stops the cough reflex. Unlike codeine, the active ingredient in most cough syrups, dark chocolate doesn't have that drowsy side effect.

8. **It's anti-aging and fights cancer**
    Dark chocolate can keep you looking young because it's packed with antioxidants, which fight toxins and free radicals in your body that cause damage to skin cells. Not only do the antioxidants slow down the aging process but they can also eliminate certain cancerous cells. Flavonols, polyphenols and proanthocyanidins are antioxidants present in dark chocolate that help slow the growth of cancer cells. Pentamer, another compound that naturally occurs in cocoa, can deactivate proteins that encourage cancer cells to continually divide.

9. **It's a mood enhancer**

It's well known that chocolate is some people's go-to food when they're feeling down. The reason is because chocolate stimulates your body's production of endorphins and serotonin, hormones that cause you to feel pleasure and happiness. Dark chocolate is also filled with phenylethylamine, the same chemical produced in your brain when you fall in love.

10. **Acts as a stress reliever**

It seems like dark chocolate is a miracle food because it can also be used to lower the risk of heart disease caused by stress. Dark chocolate helps people cope with stressful situations and feel the effect of stress less. Researchers found that people who ate dark chocolate regularly had lower levels of stress hormones, cortisol and epinephrine, circulating in their blood.

Ref: http://www.ba-bamail.com/

The Health Benefits of Eating Avocados

Smooth, creamy and flavorsome, avocados provide a unique and versatile addition to numerous dishes and snacks around the world. They can liven up a salad or soup, are the main ingredient in much-loved guacamole, and provide a fantastic dressing for any sandwich. But the avocado's unique taste and interesting texture are not the only features that ensure they stand out from other fruits. They also have an unusual nutritional make up which provide some incredible health benefits that will make you want to add them to your regular diet.

What Are Avocados

Although they are typically employed for savory uses in the kitchen, an avocado displays all the biological properties of a berry, and is classified as a fruit. Typically grown in the hot climates of Central America and the Mediterranean, they differ from other fruits not only in taste, but also due to their biological qualities. Avocados consist primarily of healthy fatty acids, rather than the carbohydrates and sugars contained within most fruits - an unusual characteristic that gives them a number of health benefits not found elsewhere.

Health Benefits of an Avocado

Numerous studies have shown that the diverse range of nutrients offered by avocados offer a wide ranging series of powerful health benefits. Here are 10 reasons to add avocados to your weekly diet, all of which have been supported by scientific research.

1. **They Contains Loads of Goodness**

    Avocados are extremely nutritious and contain abundant levels of a whole range of nutrients, including over 20 vitamins and minerals. A single, 100 gram (3.5 oz) serving of avocado will provide you with:

    - 26% of your recommended daily levels of Vitamin K, which is important for strong bones and heart health.
    - 20% of your recommended daily levels of folate, which is important for the formation of blood cells in your bone marrow.
    - 17% of your recommended daily levels of Vitamin C, which is important for supporting the immune system, heart, eyes and skin.
    - 14% of your recommended daily levels of Vitamin B5, which is important for allergy avoidance amongst other benefits.
    - 13% of your recommended daily levels of Vitamin B6, which helps various systems in the body, including the circulatory, digestive, immune, nervous and muscular systems.
    - 10% of your recommended daily levels of Vitamin E, which encourages healthy skin and eyes. In addition to these, it also contains smaller amounts of a Magnesium, Manganese, Iron, Zinc, Vitamin A and Phosphorous. Avocados really are a hotbed of essential nutrients!

2. **They Provide Friendly Fats**

    Avocados are one of the fattiest plants on the planet, but while the word 'fat' has negative connotations, not all fat is bad for you. In fact, the body needs a certain amount of 'friendly' fat to function properly. Avocados are high in polyunsaturated fats, which have been shown to reduce blood cholesterol levels and lower the risk of heart disease. Avocados are also rich in Oleic Acid, a fatty acid that is credited with providing many of the health benefits of olive oil.

3. **They Help Maintain Your Vision**

    Avocados are high in anti-oxidants including two nutrients called Lutein and Zeaxanthin, which are essential for good eye health. Studies have shown that these ingredients significantly reduce the risk of cataracts. They have also been shown to help protect you from macular degeneration, the most common cause of vision reduction or loss among people over the age of 65.

4. **They Can Reduce the Risk of Heart Problems**

    Heart disease is the most common cause of death in the western world, and there are a number of triggers that can cause it to develop. Increased levels of cholesterol and triglycerides are high on the list of common causes, and the consumption of avocados has been shown to help control levels of both. One study tested two groups of people, one group that had been instructed to eat avocados, and one group that were not. Results showed that those who ate avocados reduced blood triglycerides by up to 20% and lowered harmful cholesterol by as much as 22%.

5. **They Are Great Anti-Inflammatories**
The Omega-9 fatty acids found in avocados are anti-inflammatories, which can help balance out the negative, inflammatory effects of the unsaturated fats found in various processed foods and dairy products. They also contain high levels of nutrients called phytosterols, which also have powerful anti-inflammatory properties, and are highly recommended for people who suffer from arthritis and osteoporosis. If that wasn't enough, the phytosterols combine with oleic acid to provide proven protection against UV damage and inflammation of the skin cells. Avocados can therefore be considered something of an anti- inflammatory super-food!

6. **They Can Help Digestion**
Another nutrient avocados contain in abundance is fiber, which is associated with weight loss, blood sugar regulation and better digestion. Avocados contain an unusually high amount of fiber, with each 100 gram (3.5 oz) serving containing around 7 grams of fiber, which is 27% of the recommended daily amount. A high fiber diet can helps food pass through the digestive system more easily, maintaining the health of your colon, while reducing feelings of bloatedness.

7. **They Are A Great Source of Potassium**
Potassium takes an essential role in the generation of the electrical pulses that keep your heart beating, and also helps keep your muscles moving and your nerves working. Studies have shown that potasssium deficiences can be linked to heart problems, kidney disease and increase the risk of a stroke. Bananas are often held up as one of the best sources of potassium but guess what? Avocados contain more potassium per 100 gram (3.5 oz) - providing 14% of your recommended daily amount, compared to the 10% offered by bananas.

8. **They Help You Absorb Nutrients from other Foods**
When you eat healthy foods, it is important to ensure that your body absorbs as much of the goodness as possible, and this absorption process sometimes needs some help. Many key nutrients actually need to combine with fat to be utilized successfully, including vitamins A, D, E and K, and the hugely beneficial antioxidant Carotenoid. Carotenoids are found in leafy greens, carrots and sweet potatoes, all vegetables which contain very little fat. Studies have shown that if you add an avocado when you eat these foods, carotenoid uptake can increase up to 15 times over.

9. **They May Help Prevent Cancer**
Although research is in its infancy, there is some evidence that avocado consumption can be beneficial in preventing certain types of cancer. A 2007 study published in the journal Seminars in Cancer Biology found that phytochemicals contained with avocados could encourage cancer cells to stop growing. Other research has suggested a link between avocados and reduced risk of mouth, skin and prostate cancer. The potentially powerful benefits of avocados in this regard are linked to their unique mix of antioxidant and ant-inflammatory properties.

10. **They Can Help Regulate Blood Sugar Levels**
Because they are low in carbohydrates and sugars when compared to other fruits, avocados can help maintain blood sugar levels. Their high fiber content is also important in this regard. A large portion of any fiber-rich food eaten will pass through the the digestive system in tact, and this means they are less likely to cause a spike in blood sugar levels. People who have type 2 diabetes are often told to include plenty of fiber in the diet, and avocados are a great, source.

Sources: livescience.com and authoritynutrition.com

These are definitely NOT Brain Foods!

We've heard about foods that damage our heart, liver, and digestive system, but what about those that damage the most important organ in our body – the brain? It's more than likely that you've felt tired or groggy after eating lunch – most likely because you ate something that affected your brain in some manner. In that case, which foods should you be avoiding in order to keep your mind sharp, and which can you have in moderation?

1. **Sugar**
   It is common knowledge that large quantities of sugar are bad for you, but consuming it for a prolonged period of time may lead to neurological problems. High levels of sugar will affect your ability to learn and retain information, as well as reduce your brain's elasticity. High blood sugar levels inhibit the breakdown of insulin by the brain, leading to a reduction in mental and cognitive processes.
   Recommended daily dosage: Women – 6 teaspoons of sugar, Men – 10 teaspoons of sugar.

2. **Salt**
   Salt is known to cause problems with blood pressure, heart rate, the digestive system, and even respiratory issues. The brain uses the same cardiovascular system as these other organs, and so will be similarly damaged. Salt is essential for the body's functions, but it is highly important not to overdo it.
   Recommended daily dosage: A teaspoon of salt is the maximum recommended daily intake. For people over 50, those with diabetes or chronic kidney issues, the amount drops to half a teaspoon.

3. **Junk Food**
   There's a reason it's called **junk** food. Studies have shown that junk food can become addictive for some people. The main reason is that junk food raises the levels of dopamine in the brain (the chemical responsible for joy and satisfaction), and quitting junk food causes actual withdrawal symptoms, as well as anxiety and even depression. In increased consumption levels, it may lead to memory loss, and in rare cases it can even cause Alzheimer's.
   Recommended daily dosage: It's OK to indulge in these foods once in a while, but experts recommend that people should avoid consuming more than 500 calories in a meal. The problem is that most fast food meals contain 800 calories or more on average. Thanks to new laws, restaurants now have to display the caloric value of served food, allowing you to make sure you get the amount of calories your body truly needs.

4. **Fried food**
   Some oils, such as sunflower oil and flax seed oil, release a substance known as aldehyde. At the lowest heat level, Aldehyde is known to damage neurological brain functions. Furthermore, fried food can become addictive, similarly to junk food. Finally, a 2008 study found a correlation between the consumption of fried fish and sub-clinical disturbances in the brain, as seen in an MRI scan.
   Recommended oils for frying: While you should avoid fried food in general, if you do decide to prepare some, avoid harmful oils like sunflower and flax seed oils. Stick with healthier options such as red palm oil and avocado oil.

5. **Artificial Sweeteners**
   Aspartame is one of the most common artificial sweeteners in use nowadays, but many researchers advise to avoid it, as it may be responsible for increasing the risk of developing brain cancer. If that's not enough, artificial sweeteners lower the energy levels in the brain, and regular consumption actively slows down brain functions. These artificial sweeteners can also be found in toothpaste, processed foods, mouthwash, and even chewable vitamins.
   Recommended daily dosage: The maximum amount of sweetener, containing saccharin, an adult should consume daily is 8 sachets, which is equal to 2 cans of soft drink. As for aspartame – the maximum is higher, standing at 32 sachets, or 8 cans of soft drink.

6. **Trans Fats**
   A study on the effects of nutrition on elderly people who do not suffer from dementia, found that consumption of trans fats is linked to shrinkage of the brain, and researchers are inclined to believe that trans fats may affect the brain in a similar way to Alzheimer's. Recently, the American FDA announced that trans fats will become illegal in the United States in the near future.
   Recommended daily dosage: Experts warn about letting trans fats take up as much as 5-6% out of our total daily calorie intake. This means that if you eat around 2,000 calories a day, your trans fat intake rate should be a maximum of 0.45oz (13g). However, with recent information surfacing, it might be wise to decrease even that amount.

7. **Tofu**

   Dear vegans and vegetarians, even though tofu is considered to be a good substitute for meat, it may cause neurological issues. Researchers from Oxford University found that people between the ages of 52 and 98 who consumed large quantities of tofu were more likely to suffer from memory loss and dementia.

   Recommended daily dosage: It is recommended that you do not consume more than two cups of tofu per day.

8. **Preservatives and Processed Food**

   Preservatives, additives, food coloring and flavoring can all be found in processed and preserved foods. All of these chemicals affect our brain functions and behavior. Additionally, ingesting large quantities of these chemicals will slowly damage brain cells, causing brain shrinkage.

   Recommended daily dosage: It's hard to determine what the recommended quantities of these chemicals are, as it is always better to eat fresh foods instead. Try to avoid eating canned vegetables and fruits, as well as processed foods.

Ref: http://www.ba-bamail.com/

The Health Benefits of Pomegranate Juice

The pomegranate has been part of human history since biblical times, and is mentioned in Exodus, as well as in ancient Babylonian texts. The pomegranate is actually a berry, and each fruit contains between 200 and 1400 seeds. The pulp that covers the seeds is what we generally eat and drink, and it is very healthy!

Nutritional Value of Pomegranate:
Pomegranates are rich in ellagic acid, an antioxidant, and punicic acid, an Omega 5 polyunsaturated fatty acid that is beneficial for cell regeneration. The juice is a great source of vitamins A, C and E, and contains minerals like calcium, phosphorous, potassium and more.

Health Benefits of Pomegranate Juice:
Pomegranates have been used for their medicinal benefits throughout the Middle East and the Far East for thousands of years. The fruit contains many nutrients, such as quercetin, which helps protect the body from diabetes, cancer and heart diseases.

1. **Cardiovascular Benefits:**
   Pomegranate juice helps keep your heart healthy by assisting arterial elasticity and reducing blood-vessel inflammation. It also reduces atherosclerosis – a leading cause in heart diseases. Additionally, the juice helps in lowering the risk of arterial blockage, reducing LDL levels and increasing HDL levels.

2. **Maintains Blood Sugar Levels:**
   Despite containing fructose, pomegranate juice doesn't elevate sugar levels in the blood. Research showed that diabetics who drank pomegranate juice for 2 weeks did not experience an increase in blood sugar levels.

3. **Maintains Blood Pressure:**
   Pomegranate juice reduces lesions and inflammation in blood vessels, reducing high blood pressure. It also works as a natural aspirin, thinning the blood, improving blood flow in the body.

4. **Protection from Cancer:**
   The antioxidants in the juice eliminate free radicals, thus inhibiting cancerous cell growth. Pomegranate juice is believed to induce apoptosis – a state where cancer cells destroy themselves. It's considered highly beneficial in preventing prostate cancer, as well as blocking the hormone believed to be one of the main causes of breast cancer – aromatase.

5. **Soothes the Stomach:**
   Pomegranate juice has been used to treat diarrhea and dysentery since ancient times. It increases the production of enzymes that assist in digestion. You can add a teaspoon of honey to a glass of pomegranate juice to treat indigestion.

6. **Boosts Immunity:**
   The antioxidants in the juice stimulate white blood cells, boosting their efficiency. The juice has antibacterial and antimicrobial properties, helping to reduce mouth bacteria that causes cavities and staph infections (a group of bacteria that can cause a multitude of diseases).

7. **Prevents Anemia:**
   Anemia is caused when your body is low on red blood cells. The high levels of iron in the juice help the body produce more red blood cells. It is also considered a great remedy for red and sore eyes – simply put a few drops of the juice in your eyes.

8. **Improves Digestion:**
   When it comes to the digestive system, pomegranates work wonders in aiding the stomach and liver. It also helps soothe urinary tract infections and eases the flow of urine. Rich in dietary fiber, pomegranates help regulate bowel movements.

9. **Helps in Cartilage Regeneration:**
   Pomegranate juice is known to inhibit the enzymes that cause damage to cartilage, reducing future damage to the region. Unsweetened juice can relieve arthritis, and bone inflammation. A regular intake of juice is believed to curb the onset of Alzheimer's and other neurological issues. It is also believed to help dissolve kidney stones and even help erectile dysfunction.

10. **Anti-Aging Benefits:**
    A diet rich in pomegranate juice helps slow down aging by reducing wrinkles and fine lines caused by exposure to the sun. It also helps to sustain the regeneration of the skin, preventing hyper-pigmentation and dark spots.

11. **Suited for All Skin Types:**
The juice works wonders on dry skin, effectively penetrating the skin and moisturizing it. Punicic acid, an Omega 5 fatty acid in the juice, keeps the skin hydrated by locking in the moisture. The juice also helps reduce the production of sebum (an oily secretion of the seaceous glands), preventing outbreaks of pimples.

12. **Helps to Heal Scars:**
Pomegranate juice improves cell regeneration of the skin and can hasten the healing of wounds. The seeds themselves are also full of skin-beneficial nutrients, protecting against sunburns and healing sun-damage.

13. **Improves skin texture:**
A glass of pomegranate juice will give you fair and glowing skin. It will also prevent wrinkles by increasing the body's production of collagen, which provides support and strength to the skin.

14. **Good for Prenatal Care:**
Pomegranate juice contains many vitamins and minerals, as well as folic acid, all of which are essential in a prenatal diet. The anti-inflammatory properties help improve blood flow for both the mother and the fetus. The potassium in the juice prevents muscle cramps associated with pregnancy and is even believed to prevent premature childbirth.

15. **Pomegranate Face Mask for Glowing Skin:**
Mix 1tsp of powdered green papaya, 1tsp grape seed oil, and 1tsp grape seed extract with 2tsp of pomegranate juice, then apply to the face. Leave it on for an hour, then wash with warm water.

16. **Prevents Skin Cancer:**
The anthocyanins and tannins in pomegranate are powerful allies in the fight against skin tumors. Apply it directly to the skin and let the ellagic acid (a natural antioxidant found in most fruits and vegetables) do what it does best – inhibit the growth of cancerous cells.

17. **Prevents Hair Loss:**
Pomegranate juice strengthens the hair follicles, preventing hair loss and giving you rich, healthy hair.

Precautions:

- If you're taking blood pressure medication, the pomegranate's natural pressure-lowering abilities may result in dangerously low blood pressure.
- Do not consume pomegranate juice if you have the flu, a cough or constipation, or if you're suffering from a phlegmatic condition.
- Similarly to grapefruits, pomegranates can interfere with some types of medication, especially statins (cholesterol medicine), antidepressants, AIDS medication and narcotic pain relief medication.

Pomegranate nutritional facts:

	NUTRIENT VALUE	PERCENTAGE OF RDA
Energy	83 Kcal	4%
Carbohydrates	18.70 g	14%
Protein	1.67 g	3%
Total Fat	1.17 g	6%
Cholesterol	0 mg	0%
Dietary Fiber	4 g	11%
VITAMINS		
Folates	38 µg	9.50%
Niacin	0.293 mg	2%
Pantothenic acid	0.135 mg	3%
Pyridoxine	0.075 mg	6%
Riboflavin	0.053 mg	4%
Thiamin	0.067 mg	5.50%
Vitamin A	0 IU	0%
Vitamin C	10.2 mg	17%
Vitamin E	0.60 mg	4%
Vitamin K	16.4 µg	14%
ELECTROLYTES		
Sodium	3 mg	0%
Potassium	236 mg	5%
MINERALS		
Calcium	10 mg	1%
Copper	18%	0.158 mg
Iron	0.30 mg	4%
Magnesium	12 mg	3%
Manganese	0.119 mg	5%
Phosphorus	36 mg	5%
Selenium	0.5 µg	1%
Zinc	0.35 mg	3%

Ref: http://www.ba-bamail.com/

15 Healthy Uses For Lemons

Lemons are some of the most common citrus fruits in the world, and most of us use them almost every single day. But how much do we really know about lemons? Are we fully aware of just how beneficial they are for us, and how many other ways there are to use them, besides eating?

After reading these 15 facts and uses, you will definitely try to eat more lemons and use them in more creative ways. If you are the kind of person who never liked lemons, despite their strong taste, high vitamin C content, antioxidants, B-vitamins, calcium and more, this just might be the thing to change your mind!

Restore the pH levels in your body:

The stress of modern life, junk food, pollution, lack of exercise and other toxins we accumulate can throw our body off balance. Although lemons are very acidic, their nutrient content is alkaline-forming and thus helps make our body more resistant to a number of health problems. A cup of warm water with some lemon squeezed in will help you start your day in a healthy way.

Help your digestion process:

Lemons are powerfully antibacterial and as such they destroy bad bacteria in your body and allow good bacteria to flourish. The good bacteria help with problems such as indigestion and constipation. A glass of water mixed with the juice of one lemon, or any other means of combining lemons with a large meal, will help stimulate peristalsis and the production of stomach acids that will aid the digestion process.

A helpful dietary aid:

When you're on a diet, a lemon can be your best friend for a number of reasons. First, it contains Pectin, a fiber that can help you feel fuller and eat less. Thanks to this, a glass of lemon tea before a meal can help prevent overeating. Second, lemon juice happens to be a natural diuretic. This means it helps the body get rid of excess water it doesn't need through increased urination, this will make you feel less heavy and puffy.

Natural parasite killer:

Parasites and intestinal worms are very hard to get rid of, but there is a key element to getting rid of them that lemons contain. Parasites love acidic environments and drinking lemon juice or eating lemons will make your digestive system a more balanced environment, one that is hostile to parasites.

Natural mouth wash:

If you have bad breath or canker sores, a lemon might be an easy, cheap and simple way to deal with them. Apply fresh lemon juice to the area or gargle just like any other oral care aid. If you have bleeding gums, you can massage freshly squeezed lemon juice to the problematic area and deal with the bacteria causing all the pain directly.

Relax and increase concentration:

The gentle scent of a lemon has been scientifically proven to have a calming effect. The lemon's essential oil has the ability to increase your level of concentration and alertness while working or studying, just by enjoying the fresh scent it emits.

Exfoliate and renew your skin:

The vitamin C in lemons has a beneficial effect on your skin as well as your body. Many skin care products are high in vitamin C because it stimulates cell renewal by gently exfoliating your skin. By using a slice of lemon as a facial scrub, you will remove stubborn dirt and dead skin from your face and reveal the fresh, clean and healthy layer underneath.

Take better care of your liver:

Herbalists and naturopaths claim that the sourness of lemons signals the body to activate the liver and kidneys, and that the antioxidants in the lemon help enhance kidney and liver function. This enables them to better detoxify themselves and the rest of the body. As previously mentioned, lemons are also a mild diuretic, so they encourage your body to release stored, unused water along with the accumulated waste products flushed out by your liver.

Lower your blood pressure:

The Pectin in lemons can help lower cholesterol that causes high blood pressure. Flavonoids, as well as vitamin P, also serve to strengthen the blood vessels themselves and lower the risk of them being damaged by high blood pressure.

Keep a dandruff-free head:
A simple way to treat dandruff by yourselves is to make a hair mask using lemon juice and other natural ingredients like coconut oil. Use this mask to moisturize your dry scalp, but don't use it for too long or too often as lemon juice can also lighten your hair color.

Take better care of your feet:
The solution for rough and scaly feet might be right inside your kitchen. The citric acid along with the vitamin C in lemons can take off dead skin, enhance skin renewal, and brighten dark skin areas. Simply soak your feet in some hot water mixed with the juice of 2-3 lemons, 2 tablespoons of olive oil and ¼ cup of milk for about 20 minutes. Your feet will not only be softer than ever but will also smell much better!

A home-made cure for fever and chills:
Lemon tea and lemon juice have long been used as home-made remedies to help lower fever. A cup of lemon tea with honey every few hours should help subside any chill or fever you might have. Of course, if the fever persists - go see a doctor.

Get healthy glowing skin:
Lemons aren't just used to repair damaged skin, the high levels of vitamin C found in lemons are used by your body to make collagen and elastin. Both are tissues responsible for giving your skin a glowing and youthful appearance. Simply start eating more lemons, or apply lemon juice to your skin, and after a short while you will see the effect.

Pain relief:
The oils found in lemons create an aroma that relaxes blood vessels and reduces inflammation, both key factors in pain relief. If you suffer from sore joints or other inflammatory diseases, drink a glass of lemon water every day to help ease your symptoms. Lemon extract can even help alleviate pain caused by sunburn if applied to the skin with water and gently rubbed on the painful area.

A treatment for varicose veins:
Lemons have the ability to strengthen blood vessels, and so can be used to reduce the appearance of varicose veins, making your legs look younger and healthier. Add a few drops of lemon essential oil to a moisturizing oil of your choice (like jojoba or avocado oil) and rub the mixture onto the affected area. Doing so on a regular basis will slowly make the veins disappear from the top of your skin.

Ref: http://www.ba-bamail.com/

The Potential Risk of Grapefruit Juice

Citrus fruits are considered to be very healthy, thanks to their high vitamin C content as well as the many minerals and other nutrients they contain. However, ingesting grapefruit juice can lead to severe poisoning when mixed with certain substances. A variety of medical studies in recent years found that combining grapefruit juice with certain medications can lead to an overdose. This article will discuss the reasons for these results, and list the medications you absolutely cannot mix with grapefruit.

The Grapefruit/Medication Connection

The human body produces an enzyme called CYO3A4 that, amongst other things, helps break down certain chemicals before they are absorbed into the bloodstream. Grapefruits contain a chemical that inhibits the CYO3A4 enzyme's functions, which leads to more of the medication being absorbed into the bloodstream. When the level of medication in the blood is too high, you enter a state of overdose, which can lead to exacerbated side-effects and even poisoning.

Other Citrus Fruits

The inhibiting chemical in grapefruit can also be found in other citrus fruits, such as pomelo, limes, and bitter oranges (a type of orange that is very bitter and is mainly used in jams). It's important to mention that other species of oranges, as well as lemons - are safe to ingest, as they don't contain the aforementioned chemical.

Potential Severity of Reactions

It's difficult to predict the severity of reaction grapefruit juice will have on one's body, as it can be affected by many variables. Different juices contain different levels of the inhibiting chemical, meaning that each type of juice can have a different level of effect. Additionally, the quantity of juice consumed can have a drastically varied effect according to one's weight.

Medications that Should Not Be Taken with Grapefruit Juice:

There are currently more than 85 different medications that should not be taken with grapefruit juice, and new drugs join the list every year. The following list shows the drugs that pose the most danger when taken with Grapefruit:

Heart Rate and Blood Pressure Medication	
Generic name	Commercial names
Amlodipine	Norvasc
Amiodarone	Procor, Amiodacore, Amiocor
Felodipine	Logimax, Penedil
Nifedipine	Osmo-Adalat, Nifedipine-Teva, Pressolat, Megalat
Nimodipine	Nimotop
Quinidin	Quiniduran
Verapamil	Verapress, Apoacor, Ikacor, Ikapress, Veracor
Lipid Lowering Medication	
Generic name	Commercial names
Atorvastatin	Lipitor

| Lovastatin | Lovalip |
| Simvastatin | Simovil, Simvacor, Simvastatin-Teva |

Tranquilizers and Psychiatric Medication	
Generic name	**Commercial names**
Buspirone	Buspirol, Sorbon
Clomipramine	Anafranil, Maronil
Diazepam	Assival, Diaz, Valium
Midazolam	Dormicum, Midazol, Midazolam
Pimozide	Orap Forte
Sertraline	Lustral

Other (Immunosuppressants, antihistamines, etc.)	
Generic name	**Commercial names**
Carbamazepine	Carbi, Tegretol, Teril, Timonil
Cisapride	Prepulsid
Cyclosporine	Sangcya, Sandimmun, Deximune
Itraconazole	Sporanox
Saquinavir	Invirase, Fortovase
Sirolimus	Rapamune
Tacrolimus	Prograf

Ref: http://www.ba-bamail.com/

Eat Hummus Every Day to Reap in these Incredible Health Benefits

Hummus, a thick creamy food dip made primarily from mashed chickpeas, is both nourishing and extremely versatile - it's filling enough to be enjoyed by itself, or it can used as a spread in sandwiches or wraps.

The basic recipe contains 6 healthy ingredients: chickpeas, olive oil, garlic, lemon juice, sea salt and tahini, which have been shown to be highly anti-inflammatory, and thus can help lower inflammatory-causing chronic diseases such as rheumatoid arthritis, Alzheimer's disease, cancer, cardiovascular disease and diabetes.

Still unconvinced? Let's take a closer look at the ingredients and health benefits of hummus:

The Nutritional Facts

Hummus is packed with nutrients.
A 100g serving contains: 5g protein, 5g fiber, 9g fat, 20g carbohydrates, 13% (RDA*) vitamin c, 20% (RDA) vitamin B6, 15% (RDA) folate, 10% (RDA) iron, 10% (RDA) zinc, 11% (RDA) phosphorus, 28% (RDA) manganese.
*RDA denotes Recommended Daily Allowance

An In-Depth Look at the Ingredients in Hummus

Chickpeas: Also known as garbanzo beans, chickpeas are high in plant-based protein and fiber, which improves digestion and aids heart health. They are also exceptionally filling. Additionally, chickpeas are a good source of three nutrients that help reduce symptoms associated with PMS: magnesium, manganese and vitamin B6.

Olive Oil: In hummus, olive oil is used in its natural state. Research has shown that when heated repeatedly at a very high level, olive oil can oxidize and become hydrogenated. To prepare this recipe, opt for an extra virgin, pure olive oil free from fillers. Olive oil has been found to reduce the risk of type 2 diabetes and may help prevent strokes. It is also good for the heart. In fact, a diet rich in olive oil may slow down the aging of the heart.

Garlic: Raw garlic contains an impressive amount of nutrients, including flavonoids (plant compounds found in most fruit and vegetables). Consuming raw garlic frequently has been found to reduce risk factors associated with heart disease and various cancers. Garlic also acts as an anti-fungal, anti-oxidant, anti-inflammatory and anti-viral, and also has a number of other medicinal health benefits.

Lemon Juice: Lemons are known to have an alkalizing effect on the body, which combats high acidity levels common to most modern diets. Additionally, it helps boost immunity, digestion and helps keep blood sugar levels stable. If you're not keen on their sour taste, the health benefits lemons offer, may just change your mind.

Sea Salt: Traditional hummus uses good quality sea salt to add flavor. Himalayan sea salt in particular is a good alternative, and has numerous health benefits. It is known to keep fluid levels balanced and to keep you hydrated. Himalayan salt provides sodium levels that help balance potassium intake and they also contain important electrolytes and enzymes that aid in nutrient absorption.

Tahini

Made of ground sesame seeds, tahini offers a wide range of important micronutrients, from minerals to healthy fatty acids. Studies have shown that sesame seeds contain important beneficial properties, including antioxidant Vitamin E, and can help reduce risks associated with insulin resistance, heart disease and cancer.

While each ingredient on the list has a number of health benefits, they are especially beneficial to the body when combined in hummus. This is primarily due to the way that the fats, carbohydrates and proteins found in hummus work together. Let's take a look:

The Health Benefits of Hummus

1. **Hummus is a good source of plant-based protein**
   The main ingredient in hummus, chickpeas, provides a substantial source of protein, enabling you to feel full after consuming it. In fact you're less likely to snack in between meals due to their satiety effect. As hummus is often eaten with pita bread or other type of whole grain, it offers what is known as a 'complete protein', meaning it contains all the essential amino acids necessary for the body.

2. **It helps fight illness and disease**
    Chickpeas have been shown to help balance cholesterol levels, reduce hypertension and protect against heart disease.
    Hummus is also a good source of fiber, preventing weight gain and fat around the organs, and has been known to help
    keep the arteries clear from plaque buildup, reducing the chances of cardiac arrest and stroke. Backing this idea, studies
    have shown that a daily serving of cooked beans (3/4 cup) can help reduce chances of a heart attack and help balance 'bad'
    LDL cholesterol. Chickpeas have also been shown to have protective properties against cancer, particularly colon cancer
    - primarily because chickpeas have the ability to keep the digestive system and the colon free from harmful bacteria and
    toxic buildup. The beans found in fiber help keep waste moving out of the body quickly. Furthermore, a diet rich in beans
    has been shown to reduce hyperglycemia, helping to balance blood sugar levels. Consequently, this decreases the chance of
    developing diabetes or insulin resistance.

3. **It decreases inflammation**
    Inflammation is the body's natural defense to move toxins out. But, when your body has a high level of inflammation,
    it indicates that your body has been trying to overcome food, environmental or medicinal toxins. A diet rich in anti-
    inflammatory foods help in reducing the chance of arthritis and disease, helping to heal the body. Hummus contains both
    garlic and olive oil, both of which are anti-inflammatory foods. In one study, garlic was shown to reduce inflammation
    and help fight wrinkles and aging. Garlic has also been used to boost the immune system and cure disease, whereas olive oil
    has been found to reduce inflammation, promoting healthy cholesterol levels. What's more is that chickpeas have been
    found to reduce both inflammation and blood clots.

4. **Helps digestion and intestinal health**
    Chickpeas are an excellent source of fiber. Consequently, they help foster a healthy digestive system, making us feel full and
    satisfied for longer. Consuming enough fiber on a daily basis (about 25 to 35 grams) promotes a healthy body weight and
    decreases the chance of obesity-related diseases like type 2 diabetes, heart and many more.

5. **Hummus is high in vitamins and minerals**
    In addition to protein and fiber, hummus contains a number of essential micronutrients including iron, folate,
    phosphorus and B vitamins. The lemon juice found in hummus is also a good source of immunity boosting vitamin C
    and antioxidants. Tahini also has high levels of copper, magnesium, zinc, iron, phosphorus and calcium. Meanwhile garlic
    provides the body with manganese, vitamin B6, vitamin C and selenium, which has been shown to benefit the heart and
    boost immunity.

6. **Provides bone health**
    The sesame seeds in tahini are an excellent source of various important bone-building minerals including zinc, copper,
    calcium, magnesium, phosphorus, iron and selenium. The copper mineral found in tahini helps keep the skeletal structure
    stay strong by facilitating the binding of collagen to elastin - both of which are important building-blocks of bones.
    Calcium also helps lower levels of bone marrow loss that is typical of the aging process, and zinc has been shown to be an
    important factor in bone development and growth.

7. **Supports the heart**
    Diets rich in extra virgin olive oils help prevent cardiovascular disease in important ways. Regular consumption of good
    quality olive oil has been correlated with improving blood pressure levels, glucose, metabolism and has also been found
    to reduce cholesterol. Alongside olive oil, sesame seeds have been shown to reduce inflammation, provide important
    antioxidants and play a part in maintaining heart health by keeping the structure of arteries and cell walls healthy.

8. **Boosts your energy**
    Chickpeas contain starch, a complex carbohydrate that the body uses for energy. Starch contains natural sugars called
    glucose, which the body is able to use steadily for energy. Because starches take an extended period of time to break down,
    once consumed, your blood sugar does not spike in the same way that simple carbohydrates (flour, white bread, pasta or
    soda) can cause it to.

How to Make a Delicious Hummus

Hummus is relatively easy to make and can be prepared in under 5 minutes. The recipe below serves 8 to 10 people and can keep for up to a week in the refrigerator.

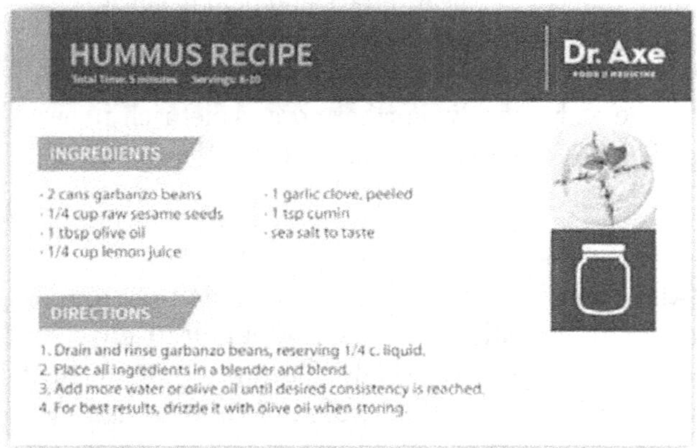

8 Nutrients You Need to Absorb Daily

Wether you're a vegetarian or meat eater, it's important to know to add certain nutritional values to your diet, or you may end up being malnurished! So, to keep your body and mind healthy, check that your daily intake covers them all!

Iodine

Iodine is essential for your metabolism, as in converting material into energy, as well as the normal functioning of the thyroid gland. It is usually found in sea fruit and so many vegetarians suffer a lack. Vegetarian sources include cooking salt, table salt and enriched dairy products.

Iron

The body requires iron to make hemoglobin which carries the oxygen in the blood stream. Red meat and poultry are a great source of iron, but if you are looking for vegetarian alternatives, you can get your iron from dried fruit, legumes, seeds, vegetables and whole wheat grains and flax seeds. Take into account that when you take these with coffee, tea or cacao, their absorption rate goes down because these products contains mixtures that block the absorption of iron. This is the reason why vegetarians are advised to consume iron with sources rich in vitamin C, such as oranges, peppers, strawberries and guavas, which markedly improve its absorption.

Omega 3

DHA and EPA are two type of the omega 3 fatty acid, and they are important to the development of both the eyes and the brain, as well as keeping your heart healthy and ticking. Omega 3 is mainly found in fatty fish, like salmon and tuna, but can also be consumed from vegetarian sources such as flax seeds, walnuts, canola oil, flax oil, soy oil and soy products. Some types of energy bars also have omega 3 in them.

Protein

Every cell in our body contains protein, and we need it in order to fix cell damage, build tissues, grow hair, fingernails and bones. Protein is in almost every food we eat, and so there's a large variety of vegetarian sources: Soy, beans, bran, lentils, chickpeas, seeds, almonds and eggs to name a few.

Calcium

Calcium, as you probably know, helps build bones and teeth (which are also bones) as well as helping the neurons in your body to transfer messages to the muscles. Fish are an excellent source of calcium, but if you're vegetarians, you can get this essential mineral from dairy products, enriched soy products, nuts, legumes and green vegetables, broccoli, okra and cabbage.

Vitamin B12

Vitamin B12 helps produce red blood cells and DNA, and is required for the neurological functioning of the body. It is found naturally in meat, but is also added to foods like soy milk and energy bars, and can also be found in eggs and various cheeses like yellow cheese, mozzarella cheese, pate cheese, cottage and eggs.

Vitamin D

Vitamin D helps the body absorb calcium and is important to bone health, as well as serving an important function in the nervous system, the muscle system and the immune system. The body makes vitamin D when the skin is exposed to the sun, but modern living as well as cloudy environments, don't always allow enough exposure. Vegetarian sources for vitamin D include: Milk and enriched soy milk, certain mushrooms, banana and avocado.

Zinc

Zinc is extremely important if you want a functioning immune system and body cells. Although it can be found a- plenty in beef, you can also consume it from soy products, peanuts, hummus, pine nuts, walnuts, almonds, wheat germ, oatmeal and a variety of legumes, if in smaller concentrations.

Ref: http://www.ba-bamail.com/

10 Amazing Spices and Herbs that Will Help you Lose Weight

Most people know that the key to weight loss lies within what you eat. What many don't know is that a key component might be collecting dust on your spice rack.

They may seem small and insignificant but spices offer much more than a kick of flavor to your meals. Many of them have ingredients that serve as potent weight loss aides when used correctly. Consider adding a natural weight loss catalyst to your diet by including some of the spices listed below into your daily routine.

1. **Ginger**

   Oils found in ginger called gingerols have antibacterial, antipyretic, and anti-inflammatory effects. A combination of vitamins and minerals make this root a health powerhouse that can also help you lose weight. It stimulates digestive enzymes to make your body absorb good nutrients quickly and avoid unhealthy ones. Studies also suggest that it may boost the metabolism to help burn off excess calories. Ginger can also be used as <u>natural medicine</u> to prevent and cure many ailments.

   Consumption: Many people stir ginger into hot liquid like tea. It's also common in extracts and herbal supplements to make it easy and convenient. Ginger is one of my most favorite herb due to its unbelievable medicinal properties and fantastic taste ! I've written on how to use ginger and other spices as medicine in my e-book **The Herbal Remedies Guide**.

2. **Cardamom**

   Cardamom has a strong smell and is widely used in the holistic Ayurveda approach to natural health for thousands of years. The spice's ability to help the digestive process and enhance metabolic function makes it ideal for weight loss. Research found that the delicious taste and smell of cardamom is also a great way to naturally alleviate depression. **Consumption**: The gently sweet and moderately smokey taste goes great in a cup of coffee, puddings, soups, potatoes, and any kind of meat to give it an Indian flair. Cardamon is also one of the ingredients in the <u>"GoldenMilk"</u> – a natural beverage that has been traditionally used to cure diarrhea, fever, bronchitis, colds and non-specific viral infections, headaches, parasitic worms, leprosy, bladder and kidney infections, and to reverse joint and muscle pain due to inflammation or arthritis.

3. **Black Pepper**

   That pepper shaker on your table might be more than just a timeless method of adding kick to virtually any dinner. A constituent called piperine, the stuff that makes you sneeze, can actually help prevent fat storage. Ui-Hyun Park of Sejong University recently found that black pepper intervened with genes in the body that create new fat cells. **Consumption**: Put it on any meat, potatoes, on your eggs, in pasta… basically any dinner dish! A simpler alternative is finding the supplements that directly release piperine into your body.

4. **Mustard**

   As a condiment mustard is one of your healthiest choices with a mere 5 calories per serving. Ingesting mustard seed is an effective way to make your body burn calories more effectively. Hot mustard is said to have the most effective thermogenic effect. Thermogenesis is the process by which the body generates heat, or energy, by increasing the metabolic rate above normal. This rise in metabolic rate is referred to as the thermogenic effect. I've already written a post about the top <u>10 foods that will increase your metabolic rate</u> which you can read to learn about other foods that have effective thermogenic effect. Mustard is one of the ingredients in my <u>cayenne warming oil recipe</u> to relieve muscle and joint pain. **Consumption**: Mustard seeds can be eaten raw but there are plenty of other ways to enjoy them. It can be sprinkled onto meat dishes, mixed into sauces, and even mixed in water with other spices like turmeric, pepper, and garlic to make your own customized condiment.

5. **Cayenne Pepper**

   Most spicy foods are associated with increasing thermogenesis. Cayenne pepper raises your temperature and as a response your body works to cool it down. This process requires your body to burn more calories as it cools. It takes only a pinch or two in your dish to give it a spicy kick as well as a healthy boost.

   Consumption: This food is great for anyone with a hankering for hot stuff. It goes well with ground meat, cooked vegetables, and is also available in powder capsules if you aren't into scorching your mouth.

6. **Ginseng**

A common ingredient to energy drinks because of its use in boosting energy and clarity. It goes beyond a mere stamina boost and also works to keep cells in your body from storing energy as fat. The release of insulin sparked from ginseng plays a crucial role in weight loss.

Consumption: The easiest way to consume ginseng is with drinks, capsules, and powder. The root can also be eaten raw or cooked, usually in a soup of some sort. The powder is commonly sprinkled on top of meats, salads, and into tea.

7. **Dandelions**

Considered a pestilent weed by many, dandelion is actually a completely edible weight loss supplement as well. It's packed with essential vitamins and minerals like calcium, potassium, and magnesium. The diuretic properties provide quick weight loss, though most of it is water weight.

Consumption: For the love of god don't scoop up a handful of flowers and eat them raw. Dried leaves and powders are commonly mixed into hot tea and other types of drinks. There's also a pill form that's easy to swallow. Fresh leaves can be added to salads.

8. **Turmeric**

Turmeric is a staple to many Indian dishes like curry and it has amazing health benefits that I've already mentioned in a previous post . It's been suggested by physicians to alleviate stress, clean the liver, lower cholesterol, and as a natural antiseptic. The curcumin in turmeric counteracts resistance of insulin in your body, making you less likely to store fat or develop diabetes. Turmeric is a true superfood that is also featured in my e-book about superfoods which is part of the **Natural Health Revolution Program**. This program will help you to achieve your health, nutrition or weight loss goals.

Consumption: Like many of the other spices turmeric can be purchased in pill and powder forms. It serves as a great addition to seafood and chicken dishes. It's also been mixed with honey and lemon to make a fat fighting tea.

9. **Cumin**

There are numerous mental and physical benefits that come from ingesting cumin. It can improve memory, concentration, prevent excessive gas and bloating and help your body absorb healthy nutrients. The high level of iron aids in healthy digestion and enhances metabolic enzymes.

Consumption: A slight nut and pepper flavor makes the cumin seed great for southern style dishes like tacos and chicken. It also goes great mixed with cooked vegetables, hot tea, and assorted beans.

10. **Cinnamon**

Cinnamon's versatility has made it a culinary staple nearly every spice cabinet. What most people don't know is the array of health benefits that come from it. Ground cinnamon is loaded with iron, calcium, fiber, and manganese. These minerals help prevent stomach ulcers, cure infection, and lower blood sugar levels. It metabolizes glucose to prevent fat storage and helps food digest in a way that makes you feel fuller for longer. Adding cinnamon to your diet is also one of the 70 habits featured in my e-book **70 Powerful Habits For A Great Health** which will guide you how to take positive steps to improve your wellness and overall health.

Consumption: Try cinnamon sprinkled in coffee, baked recipes, in hot water with honey, or on your breakfast cereal/oatmeal. Try to avoid cinnamon sugar mixes, as they contain a lot of excess calories.

Ref: May 9, 2014 Food & Nutrition Ref; Healthy and Natural World (Mr.Jenny)

20 Great Uses for Black Pepper

There's a good reason why black pepper is considered the 'king of spices'. With its aromatic taste, large selection of culinary uses, and great variety of medicinal advantages, black pepper has gained a place of honor in any kitchen or spice rack, and even in the medicine cabinet. Since ancient times, pepper appeared in many medicinal arts, for its ability to calm stomach aches, reduce liver problems, lung diseases, and digestion problems. It can also improve blood flow, act as an anti-depressant and reduce the risk of Colorectal Cancer.

My granny taught me a few great uses for this spice, and now I'll share a few with you.

1. **To keep your cholesterol low** - Add 1/4 teaspoon of black pepper to a glass of buttermilk. Mix in some finely cut onion and drink.

2. **Dealing with cold feet** - Put black pepper grains, a few pieces of garlic, and mustard seeds in a cloth bag and hang around your neck.

3. **To lose weight** - Mix 1/4 teaspoon of ground black pepper, one glass of water, 2 tablespoons of lemon juice and one of honey. Stir well and drink daily.

4. **To reduce fever** - Take 7 or 8 leaves of basil and 3 or 4 grains of black pepper and chew them together.

5. **To treat a cold** - Make some tea and add 2 or 3 grains of ground black pepper, a piece of ginger and basil leaves.

6. **To relieve a dry cough** - Grind 5 or 6 seeds of black pepper and mix with natural honey. Swallow a spoon of this mix daily until relief is achieved.

7. **To relieve asthma attacks** - Boil 8 to 10 grains of pepper, 2 clove buds and 10 to 15 basil leaves in water. Let the brew sit for about 15 minutes, strain it and add 2 spoons of honey. Tip: Drink with milk!

8. **Treating a sore throat** - Squeeze some lemon juice, add a bit of salt and ground black pepper - and gurgle.

9. **To treat a chronic cold** - Consume ground black pepper with dates.

10. **To open a blocked up nose** - Mix equal amounts of black pepper, cinnamon, cumin and cardamom seeds. Grind to a thin powder and smell or inhale the mixture. This will cause healthy sneezing and will open the nose ducts.

11. **To relieve any kind of cough** - Grind some black pepper and add sugar. Consume the mix with clarified butter.

12. **To ease a heavy cough** - add 2 or 3 grains of black pepper to a glass of boiling hot milk, wait for it to cool a bit and then drink.

13. **Treating a toothache** - Mix ground black pepper with clove oil. Smear the ointment on the afflicted area.

14. **To treat indigestion** - Mix some black pepper with ginger juice and sip after every meal.

15. **Relieve nausea** - Mix black pepper and water in a glass, add some fresh lemon juice, mix and drink slowly.

16. **Treating skin conditions** - Prepare an ointment from ground black pepper and refined butter. Apply to skin conditions such as allergy rash, Eczema and scabies.

17. **To fight baldness** - Make a thick paste from black pepper and lemon seeds. Apply it daily to balding areas about 10 minutes before showering. The solution should help revitalize hair growth.

18. **To deal with hemorrhoids** - Grind together 20 grams of black pepper, 10 grams of cumin and 15 grams of sugar. Mix in water and drink morning and evening, every day.

19. **To stop bleeding** - Cover the bleeding wound with ground black pepper. Bandage with a paper towel and tighten with cellotape (scotch tape). Wait 10 minutes and the bleeding will stop.

20. **To stop hiccups** - Hold a small plate with black pepper to your nose, inhale strongly a few times and the hiccups will cease.

Ref: http://www.ba-bamail.com/

10 Inflammatory vs. 10 Anti-Inflammatory Foods

Inflammation is a condition in which parts of the body become red, swollen, and hot. These symptoms, which are often accompanied by pain, are caused as a reaction to injury or infection. It's easy to spot inflamed areas when they are on the outside of the body. But what about internal inflammation? This can be caused by a number of reasons. One way to prevent and reduce it is to eat lots of foods that fight inflammation from within the body. For this reason, it is important to know which foods help you fight inflammation, and which are the ones that cause it.

10 foods that <u>cause</u> inflammation

1. **Sugar** - It's incredibly hard to avoid sugar - we find it everywhere. However, a lot of it may cause inflammation, so it's important to control your intake of processed sugar and opt for sweet fruit instead.

2. **Common Cooking Oils** - Safflower, soy, sunflower, corn, and cottonseed. These oils not only contribute to the onset of inflammation, but they are also made with cheap ingredients that are bad for your health.

3. **Trans Fats** - Trans fats increase bad cholesterol, and promote inflammation, obesity and resistance to insulin. They are in fried foods, fast foods, and commercially baked goods, including peanut butter and items prepared with partially hydrogenated oil, margarine, and vegetable oil.

4. **Red and Processed Meat** - Red meat contains a molecule that humans don't naturally produce, called Neu5GC. Once you ingest this compound, your body develops antibodies that may trigger constant inflammatory responses. Reduce red meat consumption and replace it with poultry, fish and lean cuts of red meat, once a week at most.

5. **Feedlot-Raised Meat** - Animals who are fed with grains like soy and corn are likely to experience inflammation. These animals also gain excess fat and are injected with hormones and antibiotics. Always opt for organic, free-range meats that have been fed natural diets.

6. **Dairy** - While some yogurts are okay, the body generally has a hard time processing dairy products. Milk is a common allergen that may cause inflammation, stomach problems, skin rashes, hives and even breathing difficulties. Remember, milk is good for children but not as great for adults.

7. **Alcohol -** Regular consumption of alcohol causes irritation and inflammation to numerous organs, which can lead to cancer.

8. **Refined Grains** - "Refined" products have no fiber and have a high glycemic index. They are everywhere: white rice, white flour, white bread, pasta, pastries... Try and replace with minimally processed grains.

9. **Artificial Food Additives** - Aspartame and MSG are two common food additives that can trigger inflammation responses. Try and omit them from your diet completely.

10. **Undiagnosed Allergy** - Do you constantly have headaches or feel tired? Sometimes, you may develop an allergy to a type of food and not even know it. Coffee, certain vegetables, cheese...they might be a trigger you aren't even aware of. Try and take a few foods out to see how you feel. Slowly incorporate them back in to see if there might be a hidden culprit lurking in your diet!

10 foods that naturally <u>fight</u> inflammation

1. **Salmon** - Salmon contains Omega 3 amino acids and has been known to treat a multitude of health issues. If you don't like eating fish, you can try a good, high-quality supplement. Try and integrate fish oil or oily fish into your meals twice a week to reap its benefits.

2. **Garlic** - Although garlic is more well-known, research is actually a bit more inconsistent about its benefits. But it can help reduce inflammation, control blood sugar and fight infections.

3. **Extra Virgin Olive Oil** - This oil has been the key to longevity in Mediterranean cultures for hundreds of years. The oil provides healthy amounts of anti-inflammatory fats and can lower the risk of asthma and arthritis, as well as protect the heart and blood vessels.

4. **Sweet Potato** - Complex carbs, beta-carotene, vitamins B6 and C, and fiber - these potatoes will work to heal inflammation raging through the body.

5. **Blueberries** - These berries not only fight inflammation, but are also excellent anti-aging agents for the brain and, above all, they fight diseases like cancer and dementia.
   Tip: Best to go for organic berries, as regular berries' small size makes it hard to wash away the pesticides.

6. **Kelp** - This brow algae extract has important roles to play in the prevention and treatment of liver and lung cancer. It's also a strong anti-inflammatory agent, anti-tumor, and antioxidant. This one does it all. Good sources for kelp are kombu, wakame, and arame.

7. **Ginger** - Regular ginger contains a multitude of potential health benefits. It fights inflammation, it helps control your blood sugar levels, and as a tea - it's really good for your diet.

8. **Turmeric** - Research is constantly mentioning the benefits of this powerful spice from Asia, which is a strong contender in the anti-inflammatory ring, thanks to its active ingredient - curcumin. This strong ingredient is believed to also fight against the development of Alzheimer's disease, counter heart problems, and act as a natural pain reliever.

Ref: http://www.ba-bamail.com/

8 Ways Coconut Water is Good for You

If there's one fruit that can bear water better than all the rest, it's the coconut. Not only could this fruit save your life when stranded on an island (though, you'll likely never come to that), it could wonderfully sustain your body with some essential nutrients as well. The liquid found beneath its thick shell is pure, potable water we can easily get our hands on from most supermarkets today. It's tastier than regular water, and it comes with these amazing health benefits too:

1. **Supports weight-Loss**
   Despite being tasty, coconut water is extremely low in fat, meaning that you can consume as much of it as you want, guilt-free. It will also make you feel fuller than the water you normally drink, because of its rich mineral content.

2. **Improves your skin's health**
   Coconut water is one of the best things you could ever give to your skin, especially if you have acne or other blemishes. In fact, we come across various skin care products that contain extracts of coconut, and now we see why. To clear up and tone your skin, simply apply some coconut water. It can even show improvements in the skin if ingested orally, as it moisturizes it from within and eliminates excessive oils.

3. **Helps in hangover recovery**
   If you've been out all night and have overdone it with alcohol, you'll find it relieving to know that you have a stock of coconut water handy in your home the next morning. It's the ultimate hangover remedy that will help settle your stomach and replace the essential electrolytes you lost in urination or vomiting.

4. **Aids digestion**
   Coconut water is also helpful when it comes to the digestion process. If you occasionally feel that you're having difficulty digesting certain foods, you're likely to feel better by drinking this water. It prevents indigestion while also reducing the occurrence of acid reflux, due to its high concentration of fiber.

5. **Promotes hydration**
   Not even sports and energy drinks are quite as good as coconut water in this regard. Compared to these popular drinks, coconut water contains double the amount of potassium (294 mg) and five times less the amount of sugar (5 mg natural sugar), per glass. Sodium count is only 25 mg, which is lower compared to the 41 mg found in sports drinks.

6. **Controls blood pressure**
   Electrolytes in food may trigger high blood pressure if found in disproportionate amounts. Coconut water contains a balanced amount of these, making it a perfect natural controller of the body's blood pressure. A good way to reap this great benefit is to drink from this water every morning.

7. **A rich source of nutrients**
   The most nutrient-rich water has got to be coconut water. The aforementioned electrolytes present in this water include calcium, magnesium, phosphorus, potassium and sodium - all of which are essential to the human body. It is also suitable for people with varying medical conditions.

8. **Compatible with human blood**
   Its incomparable taste and superb health benefits aren't the only reasons why coconut water is so widely sought after. This amazing natural beverage can be used in emergencies, as a fast way of re-hydration. It is also commonly used in poorer, third-world countries as an exceptional life-saver.

What's the recommended healthy dosage?

According to experts from the Mayo Clinic, it is recommended that consuming large amounts of coconut water should be accompanied by an active lifestyle, since each eight-ounce serving contains 45 to 60 calories. While it's good to take this advice, there's no strict rule about its consumption.

Coconut water can be enjoyed as a stand-alone beverage or even combined with other liquid products. If you're extracting it from fresh coconuts, be sure to go for the ones that are young and green, rather than the mature ones with a hard brown shell. The more mature a coconut is, the less the supply of coconut water substance it will have. To test this, you can simply shake the fruit to find out how much liquid it contains.

Ref: H/T: lifehack.org

9 Ways Neem Tree Oil Repairs Your Skin and Hair

Neem tree oil is commonly harvested from the neem tree (sometimes called an Indian lilac or by its technical name Azadirachta indica), found growing in India and other tropical regions. It is dark colored and smells like a fusion between garlic and peanuts. This healing tree oil is an important part of Ayurveda, an ancient Indian medicine practice. As a natural ingredient, it is also anti-bacterial, analgesic, anti-inflammatory and anti-fungal. It can treat many skin and hair problems.

For your skin

Protects skin from aging

Since neem tree oil is rich in antioxidants applying it to your skin can protect it from environmental damage. The oil's abundance of carotenoids can prevent free radicals from harming your skin. Neem tree oil is also rich in fatty acids and vitamins, which can improve your skin's elasticity. This helps with smoothing fine lines and wrinkles.

Clears up spotty skin

Neem tree oil can reduce the redness and inflammation caused by acne and pimples. Neem tree oil eradicates the bacteria and the concentrated fatty acids prevent acne scars from forming. Similarly applying a face mask made with neem tree oil can help get rid of any skin impurities and can help tighten your pores.

Relieves eczema

Eczema is largely a genetic disorder which causes skin abrasions, swelling and redness. Applying neem tree oil can help this disorder without having to take strong medication. The ample amounts of fatty acids and vitamin E in the oil penetrate the skin's outer layer. This provides moisture and thereby restores the protective barrier of the skin, while the antiseptic properties protect the skin from infection. There are compounds of nimbin and nimbidin in the oil, which reduce swelling and relieve the redness.

Fights fungi

Fungal infections are more widespread than most people realize. Common ones include nail fungus, ringworm and athlete's foot and can pester one to no end. Because neem tree oil is a powerful antifungal agent applying it to these infected areas can help eliminate these skin conditions quickly and naturally.

Remedies dryness

Neem tree oil is a natural skin conditioner and can help with dryness and keeping your skin moisturized. The plentiful vitamins and minerals repair any prolonged skin dryness and it's a common ingredient in moisturizing products.

For your hair

Treats head lice

Using neem tree oil is a safe alternative to the more toxic anti-lice shampoos. Applying neem tree oil won't irritate or itch your scalp while effectively killing off nits and lice. Leave neem tree oil on your head and hair overnight, and comb out the lice with a lice comb the next morning.

Promotes hair growth

Hair thinning and shedding can be caused by medication, pollution and stress. Neem tree oil has been found to be effective for people suffering from this type of hair loss. The minerals and vitamins in neem tree oil promote hair growth and can even improve the quality of your hair.

Treats split ends and frizzy hair

When your hair is weak and develops split ends it can cause hair growth to become stunted. The results are unmanageable and bushy hair. This solution also effectively helps you manage frizzy hair. Neem tree oil can make your hair more adaptable and provides a rich source of moisture, protection and works to repair damaged hair cuticles. It also makes your hair shine, and look smooth and hydrated. The best way to apply the oil is by adding a few drops to your regular shampoo. You can also apply a few drops directly to the scalp.

Treats dandruff

Using neem tree oil shampoo or a dandruff shampoo with neem tree oil can prevent and get rid of dandruff. The oil protects your scalp skin, preventing skin from shedding and maintain your scalp's PH level. The oil's rich deposits of vitamins can strengthen your hair follicles roots too.

Ref: http://www.ba-bamail.com/

10 Ways You Can Use Yogurt Other than Eat It

A cup of yogurt each morning is a great way to start the day and reap its health benefits. But this versatile dairy product has a number of other uses too, some of which extend beyond eating and drinking it. In fact, yogurt can be used as an excellent skin and hair care product, primarily due to its mild astringent qualities and its high quantities of zinc and lactic acid - making it a great, natural, hydration treatment. Best of all, it's cheap!

Let's take a look at 10 surprising uses for yogurt, you most probably, never considered:

1. **Use yogurt to lower your cholesterol**
    People with borderline to moderate-high cholesterol levels, may benefit from eating yogurt with the probiotic Lactobacillus Acidophilus, alongside a combination of the bacterium Enterococcus Faecium and Streptococcus Thermophilus. This type of yogurt is thought to lower LDL (bad) cholesterol. However, it does not raise HDL (good) cholesterol.

2. **Use yogurt to enhance your immune system**
    Yogurt contains active cultures that enhance the body's immune system. It increases the production of gamma interferons, which play a key role in fighting allergies and viral infections. Studies conducted on yogurt also found that it can help prevent gastrointestinal infections.

3. **Use yogurt to naturally whiten your teeth**
    Teeth whitening treatments are rather expensive, but why spend money when you can prepare a natural remedy with yogurt at home? Just rub some yogurt onto your teeth daily for a couple of weeks for sparkly white teeth. Yogurt is believed to work because of the phosphorus and calcium it contains.

4. **Use yogurt to relieve sunburn**
    Yogurt is a fantastic source of zinc, which helps sooth the burning and itchiness of sunburn. To relieve the symptoms, apply a thick layer of plain, cool yogurt directly to your burn and rinse off with cold water after 20 minutes.

5. **Use yogurt to relieve symptoms associated with diarrhea**
    Yogurt helps restore bacteria in the intestine, and can be used after taking antibiotics or to treat antibiotic-related diarrhea and acute diarrhea in children. In fact, a yogurt formula may be given as a replacement for milk formula in infants and young children to relieve persistent diarrhea.

6. **Use yogurt as a replacement for cheese**
    The consistency of yogurt cheese is similar to cream cheese, but is lower in fat, and contains healthy bacteria. Yogurt cheese can be used as a spread on bagels, toast and crackers and may be used as an alternative to cream cheese in cheesecake recipes. Preparing yogurt cheese is pretty simple. Empty a pint of yogurt into a large, fine-meshed strainer to catch the liquid that drains from the yogurt. The texture will vary depending on how long it drains. Then cover and refrigerate for eight to 24 hours. This will make about one cup of yogurt cheese.

7. **Use yogurt as a natural body scrub**
    Yogurt can be used as a scrub for your hands, feet or the whole body. Simply mix with oats or dried citrus peel. Massage the blend into your skin gently in a circular motion and rinse off with lukewarm water. Your skin should feel smooth and hydrated.

8. **Use yogurt as a hair conditioner**
    The properties found in yogurt make it an ideal remedy for smoothing the skin, but it's also great for your scalp and hair. Yogurt helps bring out your hair's natural shine making it soft and silky. It can be used as a hair mask instead of your conditioner. Just take some plain yogurt and rub it all over your hair, then rinse with lukewarm water. Yogurt will also help soothe an inflamed scalp, reduce hair loss and will help banish split ends.

9. **Use yogurt to relieve canker sores**
    Canker sores, white and yellow sores which usually form on your gums, inside your mouth and on your lips can be very painful to bear. Using yogurt will help reduce the pain and heal the sores. You may choose to include it in your diet or apply it directly to the affected area.

10. **Use yogurt to fight acne and prevent premature aging**
The natural antibacterial and antifungal properties found in yogurt can be used to get rid of pimples. Apply the yogurt to acne prone areas and let it sit for 30 minutes, then wash off with lukewarm water. The lactic acid found in yogurt helps dissolve dead skin and can be used to prevent wrinkles and fine lines as we age.

Ref: http://www.ba-bamail.com/

20 Foods that will Naturally Lower Your Blood Pressure

After being diagnosed with high blood pressure, alongside taking my medication, I started incorporating more of these foods into my daily meals. In the process, I discovered that eating a healthy diet rich in whole grains, fruits, vegetables and low fat dairy have kept my cholesterol levels and blood pressure levels in check. Here are 20 power foods that will lower your blood pressure naturally.

1. **Peas**
Peas are a good source of vitamins and folic acid, providing overall cardiovascular support, making them a perfect food to prevent high blood pressure.

2. **Potatoes**
Although potatoes are known to be high in starch, more evidence is pointing to their beneficial properties when consumed in reasonable amounts. UK scientists believe that a compound found in potatoes, known as kukoamine, may potentially lower blood pressure.

3. **Celery**
Celery can help your heart and your veins function better. Consequently, celery can help keep your blood pressure levels in check.

4. **Green Beans**
Green beans are a good source of vitamin C, fiber and potassium - all of which can lower your blood pressure.

5. **Papaya**
Papaya is a fantastic source of vitamin C. It also contains a large quantity of amino acids and is rich in potassium - all contributing to a healthy heart and lower blood pressure levels.

6. **Oats**
Start your morning off with a healthy bowl of oatmeal - a fantastic option to keep your blood pressure in check. Be sure to stay away from flavored types that contain sugar, as it will only raise your blood glucose levels and negate some of the effect.

7. **Yogurt**
Yogurt is a good source of potassium, magnesium and calcium - three nutrients that enable you to keep your fat content low, which in turn may help keep your blood pressure in check. To get the most out of the health benefits of yogurt, combine it with one of the foods on this list.

8. **Tomatoes**
Blood pressure is one of the things tomatoes have been shown to help with. To get the most of tomatoes, it is best to eat them close to raw, without much processing or cooking.

9. **Kiwi**
Research has shown that eating three kiwis a day can help keep your blood pressure from becoming a problem. Though this may not seem convenient, alternatively, you may pair one kiwi with other foods on this list - particularly those rich in antioxidants.

10. **Blueberries**
Like raspberries, blueberries are packed with antioxidants, which in turn have a direct impact on your blood pressure. For a nutritious breakfast and a healthy start to your day, combine blueberries with other foods that combat high blood pressure.

11. **Spinach**
Spinach is packed with nutrients and contains antioxidants helping your body repair damage from free radicals, often caused by stress. Add it to a smoothie, giving your body a boost in lowering your blood pressure.

12. **Avocados**
Avocados help fend off high blood pressure in many ways. They are a good source of potassium, fiber and are high in monounsaturated fats, all of which will help keep your blood pressure stabilized.

13. Prunes

Studies show that prunes are especially good for the body, particularly in maintaining blood pressure. They are knows to significantly reduce LDL 'bad' cholesterol in the body, hence lowering blood pressure, and are also a good source of fiber, relieving constipation.

14. Carrots

Carrots contain antioxidants and are also a good source of potassium - two major supporters of normal blood pressure levels.

15. Wild Salmon

Wild salmon contains omega-3s which prevent the blood from clotting, thus improving the circulatory system. Wild salmon is also thought to ward off heart attacks, making it an excellent food for keeping your blood pressure in check.

16. Watermelon

Watermelon contains L-citrulline, which helps relax your arteries, thus lowering blood pressure levels.

17. Raisins

Snack on raisins between meals to reap their health benefits. They are a fantastic source of potassium - just be sure to get the raw, natural kind, without added sugar.

18. Dark Chocolate

The antioxidants found in good-quality dark chocolate can help fend off free radicals, thus controlling blood pressure. Just be sure to control your portions, limiting your daily intake.

19. Beans

It has long been known that beans are excellent at balancing blood sugar levels. Adding to this, however, recent findings have also suggested that beans have a positive effect on blood pressure levels.

20. Spices

Keeping your blood pressure down does not mean that you need to sacrifice flavor. Several spices are known to keep the body in a relaxed state, helping your circulatory system to function optimally.

Ref: http://www.ba-bamail.com/

Apple Cider Vinegar is Not Just for Food

Apple Cider Vinegar is often used for salad dressings, marinades, vinaigrettes, and chutneys, but that's not all: It's also known to prolong the feeling of satiety after eating, it has well-documented anti-glycemic effects, and quite a few other uses that everyone should know about.

1. **Detox Tea**

2. **Varicose Veins Remover**

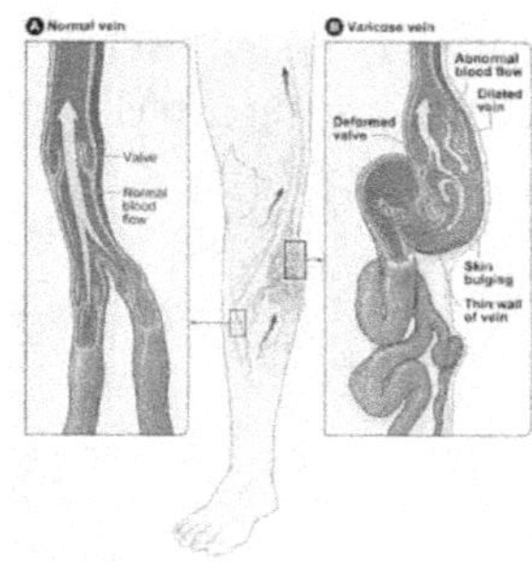

Rub apple cider vinegar onto your veins twice a day, and drink a teaspoon once a day.

3. **All-Natural Toner**

4. **Get Rid of Warts**

    What you need:

    - Apple cider vinegar
    - Cotton wool
    - Medical tape

    What you do:

    1. Clean the area.
    2. Fully soak the cotton wool with apple cider vinegar.
    3. Place the soaked wool on the wart and cover with medical tape (or bandage).
    4. Repeat daily until the wart dries out and falls off (should take up to a week).

5. **Treat Nail fungus**
    Soak your toenail in a 1:2 solution of vinegar and water for 15 minutes a day.

6. **Chemical-Free Flea & Tick Repellant**
    Make a 1:1 solution of water and **organic** apple cider vinegar in a spray bottle, and spray the dog once a week. If your dog doesn't like being sprayed, use a soaked washcloth instead. You can also add a teaspoon of organic apple cider vinegar to the dog's water twice a week for similar results. Be sure to use **organic**ACV, as the more processed kind is not good for dogs.

7. **Say "Bye Bye" to Moles**

    What you need:

    - Organic apple cider vinegar
    - Sterile needle (use rubbing alcohol or fire to sterilize it)
    - Cotton wool

    What to do:
    1. Clean the area.
    2. Use the sterile needle to poke a few holes in the mole. (There are no nerves, so it won't hurt).

3. Apply an ACV-soaked piece of cotton to the mole for 20-30 minutes.
4. Repeat daily until the mole falls off. (Should be within a a week).

8. Effective Fruit Fly Trap

What you need:

- A jar
- Raw apple cider vinegar
- Small piece of paper
- Liquid dish detergent

What to do:

1. Mix 2/3 cup of apple cider vinegar and about a tablespoon of dish detergent in a jar.
2. Create a cone out of the piece of paper and put it in the jar, as shown in the picture.
3. Leave the jar where the fruit flies are and let the mix work its magic.

9. Homemade Weed Killer

Mix ½ gallon (2 liters) of apple cider vinegar, ¼ cup salt, and ½ teaspoon of liquid dish detergent. Put in a spray bottle and spray any weed you want to get rid of.

10. Homemade Cough Remedy

What you need:

- 2 tablespoons of apple cider vinegar
- 2 tablespoons of honey
- 2 tablespoons of water
- ¼ teaspoon of cayenne pepper
- ¼ teaspoon of ground ginger

What to do:

Mix all the ingredients in a jar and shake well. Take a teaspoon for a child aged 2-9 years, and a tablespoon for ages 10 and up.

11. Better Hair Care With Baking Soda and ACV What you need:

- Apple cider vinegar
- Baking soda
- Water
- Squeeze bottle

What to do:

Hair wash:

1. Mix 4-5 tablespoons of baking soda with 1 cup of water and pour into a squeeze bottle.
2. Wet your hair, then pour the mixture on it. Make sure to get it on all of your hair.
3. Let it sit for about a minute, then rinse thoroughly.

Conditioning:

1. Make a mixture of 1:4 ACV and water.
2. Squeeze any excess water from your hair.
3. Cover your hair with the mixture and rub it in as you would with regular conditioner.
4. Thoroughly rinse your hair.

12. **Soothe and Heal a Sunburn**
   Apply straight to the burn, or you can dilute it with a bit of water if it stings too much. Use a towel or washcloth and keep it on the affected for 20-30 minutes.

13. **Heal Eczema**
   Mix ¼ cup of apple cider vinegar with 3 cups of water and lightly apply on the affected area. Caution – it may sting. H/T: *diply.com* / Title photo: *flickr.com*

Ref: http://www.ba-bamail.com/

Regular Vs Diet Soda - Which Is Worse?

It's well documented that both soda and diet soda are bad for the health, yet many of us can't resist them altogether and prefer to choose the 'lesser evil'. However, the question of which of the two is the 'lesser' evil is debatable, and indeed diet varieties can be equally as damaging as regular soda, just in different ways. Here's a breakdown of the difference between regular and diet soda that will help you make an informed decision next time you pick up that soft drink.

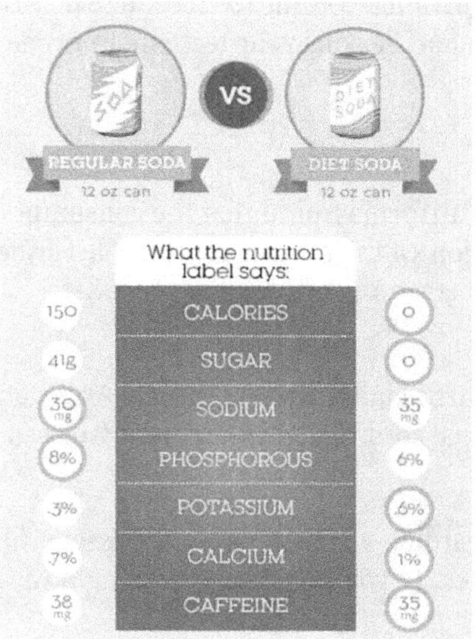

Diabetes

Regular Soda
An average can of a soda such as Coke contains nearly 10(!) teaspoons of sugar. If you consume 1-2 daily, you increase your risk of becoming diabetic by 26%.

Diet Soda
While diet varieties are preferable for diabetics, studies have shown that consuming artificial sweeteners can exacerbate a diabetic state by increasing the body's glucose intoleranc

Weight

Regular Soda
A single can of soda contains almost twice the daily recommended intake of sugar. By drinking one can per day, you'll gain an extra 2-7kg (4.5-15.5lbs) a year. In addition to this, you are consuming 'empty' calories which do nothing to satisfy your hunger so you will still want to eat afterwards.

Diet Soda
Studies have shown that even so-called diet sodas can lead to weight gain when consumed without a diet plan or regular physical exercise. The artificial sweeteners cause our brain to want more sugar, making it search for the 'real thing'.

Heart Diseases

Regular Soda
A 2012 study found that drinking one can of soda every day can increase your risk of a heart attack by 20% when compared to people who don't drink it at all. Additionally, the study found that the more sodas you drink, the more you put yourself at risk of developing obstructive lung disease associated with asthma and smoking.

Diet Soda
In several studies comparing people who drank diet soda daily, against people who didn't drink soda at all, it was discovered that diet soda drinkers are 50% more likely to develop cardiovascular problems, leaving them more prone to heart conditions and strokes. A separate study also concluded that daily consumption of diet soda raises your risk of developing cardiovascular diseases by 48%.

Oral Health

Regular Soda

Ordinary sodas contain acids that dissolve the enamel of your teeth and lead to tooth decay, plus the bacteria in our mouth thrive on the sugar. This is why drinking soda is double-trouble for your teeth.

Diet Soda

Many of you may think that diet sodas aren't harmful to your teeth because they don't contain sugar. However, they do contain phosphoric acid, which damages protective enamel, leaving your teeth more prone to attack from harmful bacteria.

Neurological Effects

Regular Soda

In 2002, researchers from the University of California found that the consumption of high levels of processed sugar - the same kind found in soda - can decrease the production of the protein responsible for neural development, causing 'Brain-derived Neurotrophic Factor', which affects memory creation and learning processes.

Diet Soda

Studies conducted as early as 1987 found that artificial sweeteners, such as Aspartame (which is used in Diet Coke), are harmful to the neural nervous system, as well as the spinal cord. These sweeteners have been associated with mood swings and headaches.

Conclusions

It's hard to reach a definitive conclusion regarding which soda is the 'lesser evil', as both present their own health problems and it is difficult to find any benefits of either. If you only take one thing away from this comparison, it's this: <u>You shouldn't be drinking either of them.</u>

That said, if you are diabetic, diet soda is the preferred drink of the two, as long as you limit yourself to no more than a few cups each month and avoid other sugary foods. If you're not worried about your weight and prefer to avoid the damages artificial sweeteners cause, stick to regular soda, but don't consume it in large quantities.

If you truly want to stay healthy, abandon sodas altogether and substitute them with natural juices, plain soda water, or a healthy, fruit-infused drink.

Ref: http://www.ba-bamail.com/

Surprising Ways Onions Can Be Used As a Medicine

The onion is a staple ingredient of a whole variety of dishes around the world. However, it also offers a wealth of health benefits that most people don't know about. Its medicinal qualities have been recognized for centuries and it has been used for its healing powers by a number of cultures and civilizations. If you didn't already know about the incredible healing powers of the humble onion, then prepare to be amazed!

Onions as Part of Your Diet

There are many good reasons why onions should be used as part of your diet. Studies into its nutritional value have concluded that they have a number of health benefits and are effective in:

- Lowering your susceptibility to Colon Cancer
- Lowering your susceptibility to Prostrate Cancer
- Lowering your susceptibility to Stomach Cancer
- Helping your sleep patterns and improving your mood
- Providing strength and structure for your skin and hair

Onions can be incorporated into a wide variety of dishes, so it is easy to fit them into a weekly dietary plan. Eating onions just two or three times a week can make a big difference. However, including them in your diet is not the only way you can use onions to postively affect your health. They have a number of medicinal and healing properties that can be used to fight various ailments. We fully expect some of them to surprise you!

Which Properties of an Onion Make It Such an Effective Healer?

Onions are packed full of a compound called Quercetin which has both strong anti-bacterial properties and the ability to fight harmful toxins. It is a powerful antihistamine, anti-inflammatory and a lowerer of cholesterol levels. The densest concentration of Quercetin is found in the outer rings nearest to the bulb's skin as well as the part of the onion that is closest to the root. This goodness is found in both red and white onions, and both types can be used as part of these natural remedies.

1. **Onions Can Heal Cuts**

   Onions are effective in the treatment of cuts to the skin. If you nick yourself with a knife cutting one, try applying a slice of the onion to the injured area immediately. The raw onion will prevent infection and clean the wound. Next, take a piece of the onion's skin and place it over the top of the wound, sealing it with an adhesive. You should find the bleeding stops quickly and the wound looks clean. If you have a larger cut or graze, use gauze to fix a piece of onion over the top of it. You can keep the onion on the wound for as long as required, just make sure you change the gauze regularly.

2. **Onions Can Lower a Fever**

   Here's an odd one for you, but an onion in a sock is a surprisingly successful means of lowering your body temperature when you are suffering from a high fever! Chop up some potatoes and slice an onion in half. Put one half of the onion into one sock, and the other half into the other (with some potato slices in each of the socks as well). Next, put the socks on your feet trying to ensure that the mixture is pressed against your soles. You should find that your temperature lowers in a relatively short time - it might sound crazy but there are many examples of success stories!

3. **Onions Can Cure Earache and Help Remove Wax**

   An onion's anti-inflammatory properties make it a powerful defense against earache and they can also be used to soften ear wax, making the wax easier to remove. If you are suffering from an earache, chop up an onion, take the inner part (that is the hard section at the 'heart' of the onion) and place it in your ear for remedial relief. You will achieve best results by completing the procedure shortly before you got to sleep. If you are someone who suffers from regular, excessive wax build-up, then you might want to perform this trick regularly.

4. **Onions Can Fight the Common Cold**

   One of the oldest recognized uses of an onion is its employment as a weapon to fight the common cold. If you feel you are developing the tell-tale signs of a coming cold (sniffles, sore throat etc) then raid your cupboard for an onion. It is most effective when eaten raw, and you should try and eat a whole one (perhaps chop it up and mix it in a salad to make to the process more palatable). Alternatively, boil the onion and use it alongside ginger and honey to make a tea. It will raise your defenses and help you fight off the cold.

5. **Onions Can Sooth Burns**

Onions are incredibly effective in soothing small burns and the recipe for doing so could not be simpler. If you have burnt yourself in the kitchen or garage, simply take half a chopped onion and apply it directly to the wound. Hold it in place for a few minutes and the pain should quickly start to ease. For further relief, whip up two or three egg whites in a bowl and use them to cover the affected area. Hold the mixture in place using a breathable bandage and you will have a natural, protective layer that will quicken your recovery.

6. **Onions Can Provide Cough Relief**

The use of onions as part of a cheap, effective cough remedy is another practice which dates back centuries. It is best employed with a few other basic ingredients and there are a couple of things you can try. Firstly, you can peel a red or white onion, and cut it into large slices. Layer the slices in a sealable jar and place brown sugar on top. Close the lid of the jar and let it sit for some time (around 6 hours is optimum). A syrup will form in the jar. Take a spoonful of the syrup as regularly as needed. The brown sugar makes the syrup more palatable and the resulting mixture does not taste too bad. Re-make the syrup every couple of days, replacing the old mixture with new. If you want an alternative, pour honey over the sliced onion instead of the brown sugar (use both if you have a particularly sweet tooth). Add a sprinkling of grated garlic for an extra health boost.

7. **Onions Can Remove Eye Irritations**

An onion's ability to remove eye irritants is derived from its most widely known feature - its ability to make our eyes water when chopped. This is a great property if you need to form some liquid in your eye to flush out an unwanted bit of dirt, a pesky fly or any other small irritant before it turns your whole eye red. Simply chop an onion and let nature takes its course! It is important you make sure you don't touch your eye after chopping the onion though - that will add to your pain. Wash your hands thoroughly before you do so.

8. **Onions Can Fight Insect Stings**

Here is where the antihistamine properties of an onion come in handy. If you are stung by a bee or wasp, then a bit of crushed or grated onion applied directly to the skin can be extremely beneficial for pain relief. The antihistamine will prevent an allergic reaction while the anti-inflammatory qualities of the onion will reduce any associated swelling. Keep the onion in place until the pain has subsided by using a breathable bandage that you should replace regularly.

Sources: healthyfoodhouse and vintageamanda

The Incredibly Nutritious Health Benefits of Eggs

Besides being an incredibly versatile ingredient that can be used in most dishes - savory or sweet - eggs are exceptionally nutritious. Their goodness can be found in the yolk, which contains over 90 percent of an egg's calcium and iron, while the white part contains almost half of the egg's protein.

So, if you're not eating eggs regularly, here are 10 reasns you ought to change your mind.

1. **They are among the most nutritious food on the planet.**

   Eggs contain a little bit of almost every nutrient we need, making them the perfect food. In fact, a single boiled egg contains:

   - Vitamin A (6% of the RDA*)
   - Folate (5% of the RDA)
   - Vitamin B5 (7% of the RDA)
   - Vitamin B12 (9% of the RDA)
   - Vitamin B2 (15% of the RDA)
   - Phosphorus (9% of the RDA)
   - Selenium (22% of the RDA)

Eggs also contain decent amounts of Vitamin D, Vitamin E, Vitamin K, Vitamin B6, Calcium and Zinc.
Intotal, eggs equate to 77 calories, 6 grams of protein and 5 grams of healthy fats.

***RDA** - Recommended Daily Allowance

2. **While eggs may be high in cholesterol, they don't adversely affect blood cholesterol.**

   True, eggs are high in cholesterol. In fact, a single egg contains 212mg, which is over half of the recommended daily intake of 300mg. However, while it may seem counter-productive to eat eggs, the cholesterol in eggs does not necessarily raise cholesterol in the blood. Of course, it is important to note that the response of egg consumption varies from one individual to another. But overall, studies have shown that in 70 percent of people, eggs did not raise cholesterol at all. However, in the other 30 percent (termed hyper responders) eggs mildly raised total and LDL cholesterol.

3. **For the most part, eggs actually raise HDL (Healthy) Cholesterol.**

   Often termed the good cholesterol, consuming eggs are a great way to increase HDL. In one study, it was found that those who consumed two eggs per day for six weeks, saw their HDL increase by 10 percent. It has also been shown that people with higher levels of HDL, usually have a lower risk of heart disease, stroke and various health problems.

4. **Eggs contain Choline - an incredibly important nutrient that most people do not get enough of.**

   This important nutrient is grouped within the B vitamins. It is used to build cell membranes and plays a role in the production of signaling molecules in the brain. However, according to dietary surveys, 90 percent of the U.S population is getting less than they ought to. Whole eggs are therefore an excellent source of choline, as a single egg contains more than 100mg.

5. **Eggs convert LDL Cholesterol particles from small and dense to large. This change in particles has been linked to a reduced risk of heart disease.**

   It is a well known fact that having high levels of LDL (bad cholesterol) is linked to an increased risk of heart disease. However, what is not well known is that there are subtypes of LDL. See, there are small, dense LDL particles, and there are also large LDL particles. Studies have shown that people who predominantly have small, dense LDL particles also have a higher risk of heart disease than those with large LDL particles. So, as I pointed out in the third fact, while eggs may mildly raise LDL cholesterol in some individuals, studies have shown that eggs may potentially change LDL particles from small and dense to large.

6. **Two of the antioxidants found in eggs (Lutein and Zeaxanthin) are beneficial for eye health.**

   Ageing usually brings with it the onset of poorer eyesight. Thankfully though, several nutrients can help counteract some of the degenerative processes which can affect our eyes. Lutein and Zeaxanthin are two such powerful antioxidants which tend to build up in the retina of the eye. In a controlled trial, it was found that eating 1.3 egg yolks per day for 4.5 weeks increases blood levels of Lutein (by 28 to 50 percent) and Zeaxanthin (by 114-142 percent). Furthermore, studies have shown that consuming adequate amounts of these nutrients can significantly reduce the risk of cataracts and macular degeneration - two very common eye disorders. Eggs also contain substantial amounts of Vitamin A, which can reduce blindness.

7. **Eggs rich in Omega-3, lower triglycerides (a risk factor for heart disease).**
   Not all eggs are created equal. Their nutrient composition varies depending on what the hens were fed and how they were raised. Hens that were raised on pasture and/or fed Omega-3 enriched foods tend to lay eggs that have a much higher Omega-3 fatty acids content - a nutrient that is known to reduce blood levels of triglycerides (a risk factor for heart disease).

8. **Eggs are a great source of protein - the main building blocks of the human body.**
   Ensuring that you get enough protein in your diet is important - in fact, it has been suggested that the Recommended Daily Amounts (RDAs) may be too low. But, seeing that eggs contain all the essential amino acids in the right ratios, our bodies are easily able to absorb the protein found in eggs. Eating adequate amounts of protein may also help with weight loss, increasing muscle mass, lowering blood pressure and optimizing bone health. One single, large egg contains **6 grams** of protein.

9. **Eggs may actually reduce the risk of a stroke.**
   Eggs have been unfairly demonized for decades, due to the levels of cholesterol found in them. However, many studies have examined the relationship between egg consumption and the risk of heart disease. In one meta-review of 17 studies, with a total of 263,938 participants, no association was found between egg consumption and heart disease or stroke. However, some studies have found that people with diabetes who ate eggs can have an increased risk of heart disease. Nevertheless, whether the eggs are actually causing the increased risk is not known.

10. **Eggs score high on the Satiety Index, inducing feelings of fullness and reducing subsequent calorie intake.**
   Eggs are high in protein, which is one of the most fulfilling macronutrients. In one study of 30 overweight women, it was found that eating eggs instead of bagels for breakfast, increased feelings of fullness, making them automatically eat fewer calories during the following 36 hours. It was also found that eating an egg for breakfast caused significant weight loss over a period of 8 weeks.

Ref: http://www.ba-bamail.com/

Health Benefits of Common Herbs & Spices

We all like to add herbs to our food. They can improve its taste and give a dish that extra little something it was missing. In addition to these great advantages, did you know that most herbs and spices also have amazing health benefits?

Chives

Low in calories (100 grams of it contain only 30 calories), chives are rich in dietary fiber, with 100 grams containing 7% of your daily intake. Chives are also rich in antioxidants, such as allicin, which is shown to reduce cholesterol production and has anti-fungal, anti-bacterial and anti-viral properties. Allicin also helps reduce blood pressure and helps prevent strokes, coronary artery disease, and peripheral vascular diseases.

Chives also contain vitamin A and antioxidants, such as carotenes, zea-xanthin, and lutein, which together offer the human body protection from lung and oral cancer. Furthermore, chives are one of the best sources for vitamin K in nature, which helps limit neuronal damage in the brain and is essential for the treatment of Alzheimer's.

Packed with minerals such as copper, iron, manganese, zinc and calcium, these leafy greens contain several vital vitamins such as B-6, B-5, B-3, B-2, and B-1 in healthy proportions.

Cilantro

Cilantro contains many antioxidants, essential oils, vitamins and dietary fibers that help reduce bad cholesterol (LDL) and raise good cholesterol (HDL). The leaves and seeds contain oils such as borneol, linalool, cineole, cymene, terpineol, dipentene, phellandrene, pinene, and terpinolene, and the stems are rich in polyphenolic flavonoids (such as quercetin, kaempferol, rhamnetin, and epigenin). Cilantro is a good source of minerals like potassium, calcium, manganese, iron and magnesium, which help control heart rate and blood pressure. It is also rich in many vitamins like folic acid, B-2, B-3, vitamin A, beta-carotene and vitamin C (all are essential to your health). Some 100 grams of cilantro leaves provide you with 30% of the daily recommended levels of vitamin C (a powerful antioxidant). Vitamin A is required for maintaining skin and mucous membrane health. It is also essential for vision, and like chives, cilantro is also rich in vitamin K.

Basil

Basil contains oils such as eugenol, citronellol, linalool, citral, limonene and terpineol, which have anti- inflammatory and anti-bacterial properties. Basil is very rich in beta-carotene, vitamin A, cryptoxanthin, lutein and zea-xanthin. These help protect against free radicals (that play a role in aging and various disease processes). Zea-xanthin was found to filter harmful UV rays and protect your eyes' retinas.

Basil contains a good amount of minerals like potassium, manganese, copper, and magnesium. All help to control heart rate and blood pressure. Basil leaves are an excellent source of iron - a component of hemoglobin inside your red blood cells.

Dill

Dill sprigs and seeds contain many essential oils (d-carvone, dillapiol, DHC, eugenol, limonene, terpinene and myristicin) and have been used as a local anesthetic and anti-septic. Dill was also found to reduce blood sugar levels in people with diabetes. Oil extracted from the seeds has anti-spasmodic, carminative, digestive, disinfectant and sedative properties, and is rich in B-9, B-2, B-3, vitamin A, beta-carotene and vitamin C.

Dill is a great source of minerals such as copper, potassium, calcium, manganese, iron, and magnesium. Copper is essential for many of the body's vital enzymes (like cytochrome c-oxidase and superoxide dismutase).

Zinc is an essential component in many enzymes that regulate the body's growth and development, sperm production, digestion and nucleic acid synthesis. Potassium is important for cell and body fluids that assist with controlling heart rate and blood pressure. Manganese is essential for the antioxidant enzyme, superoxide dismutase.

Thyme

Thyme has disease-preventing and health-promoting properties. It contains thymol, an essential oil, which has been found to have antiseptic and anti-fungal characteristics. Thyme contains flavonoid phenolic antioxidants, like zea-xanthin, lutein, pigenin, naringenin, luteolin, and thymonin.

Thyme leaves are one of the best sources of potassium, iron, calcium, manganese, magnesium, and selenium, and are a rich source of many important vitamins such as B-complex vitamins, beta- carotene, vitamin A, vitamin K, vitamin E, vitamin C and B-9.

Thyme provides about 27% of our recommended daily intake of vitamin-B-6 - a beneficial neurotransmitter for the brain, that helps with reducing stress. Fresh thyme is one of the richest in antioxidant among all herbs.

Turmeric

Turmeric has been in use since ancient times. Known for its anti-inflammatory, carminative and anti- microbial properties, it also contains essential oils such as termerone, curlone, curumene, cineole, and p-cymene.
Curcumin is the pigment that gives turmeric its orange color. Studies suggest that the curcumin may have anti-tumor, anti-oxidant, anti-arthritic, anti-amyloid, anti-ischemic, and anti-inflammatory properties. Turmeric is rich in antioxidants and dietary fiber, which help control bad cholesterol levels.
Turmeric is a rich source of many vitamins such as B-6, choline, B-3, B-2 and more. B-6 is used in the treatment of CBS deficiency, anemia and even radiation sickness. B-3 helps prevent dermatitis, and B-2 helps the body convert carbohydrates into sugar, which in turn gives us energy.
Fresh turmeric root contains high levels of vitamin C, which helps the body develop immunity against infections and remove harmful free radicals. Turmeric also contains healthy amounts of minerals like calcium, iron, potassium, manganese, copper, zinc and magnesium.

Rosemary

Rosemary leaves contain certain phytochemicals that are known to have disease-preventing and health- promoting properties. The herb parts, (especially the flower tops) contain phenolic antioxidant rosmarinic acid, as well as numerous oils that are beneficial to human health, such as cineol, camphene, borneol, bornyl acetate, alpha-pinene, and more. These compounds are known to reduce irritations and inflammations, as well as for having anti-fungal, antihistaminic and antiseptic properties.
Rosemary contains very good amounts of vitamin A, and is exceptionally rich in many B-complex groups of vitamins, such as B-9, B-5, B-6, and B-2. It also contains high levels of folates, which are important for DNA synthesis.
Fresh rosemary leaves are a good source of vitamin C, which is required for collagen synthesis in the body (collagen is required for maintaining the integrity of blood vessels, skin, organs, and bones). Regular consumption of foods rich in vitamin C protects the body from scurvy, boosts its immunity and helps clear it of free radicals.
Fresh or dried, rosemary is a rich source of minerals like potassium, calcium, iron, manganese, copper, and magnesium, and it is an excellent source of iron (a component of hemoglobin inside red blood cells, which determines the oxygen-carrying capacity of the blood).

Parsley

Parsley contains essential oils like myristicin, limonene, eugenol, and alpha-thujene, as well as flavonoids, including apiin, apigenin, crisoeriol, and luteolin. Many of these (particularly myristicin) have been shown to inhibit the formation of tumors in the lungs.
Myristicin also activates the enzyme glutathione-S-transferase, which helps attach the molecule glutathione to oxidized molecules that can be very harmful to the body. The oils in parsley qualify it as a "chemoprotective" food, meaning it can help neutralize particular types of carcinogens.
The flavonoids in parsley (especially luteolin) function as antioxidants, halting the damage that free radicals cause to the body. Additionally, extracts from parsley will help increase antioxidant capacity in the blood.
Parsley is an excellent source of vitamin A and vitamin C, and is helpful with preventing recurrent ear infections and colds. Beta-carotene (another important antioxidant in parsley), is known to reduce risk of the development and progression of certain conditions, such as diabetes, atherosclerosis and colon cancer. It may also help with reducing asthma attacks and some forms of arthritis.

Ref: http://www.ba-bamail.com/

Common Health Issues

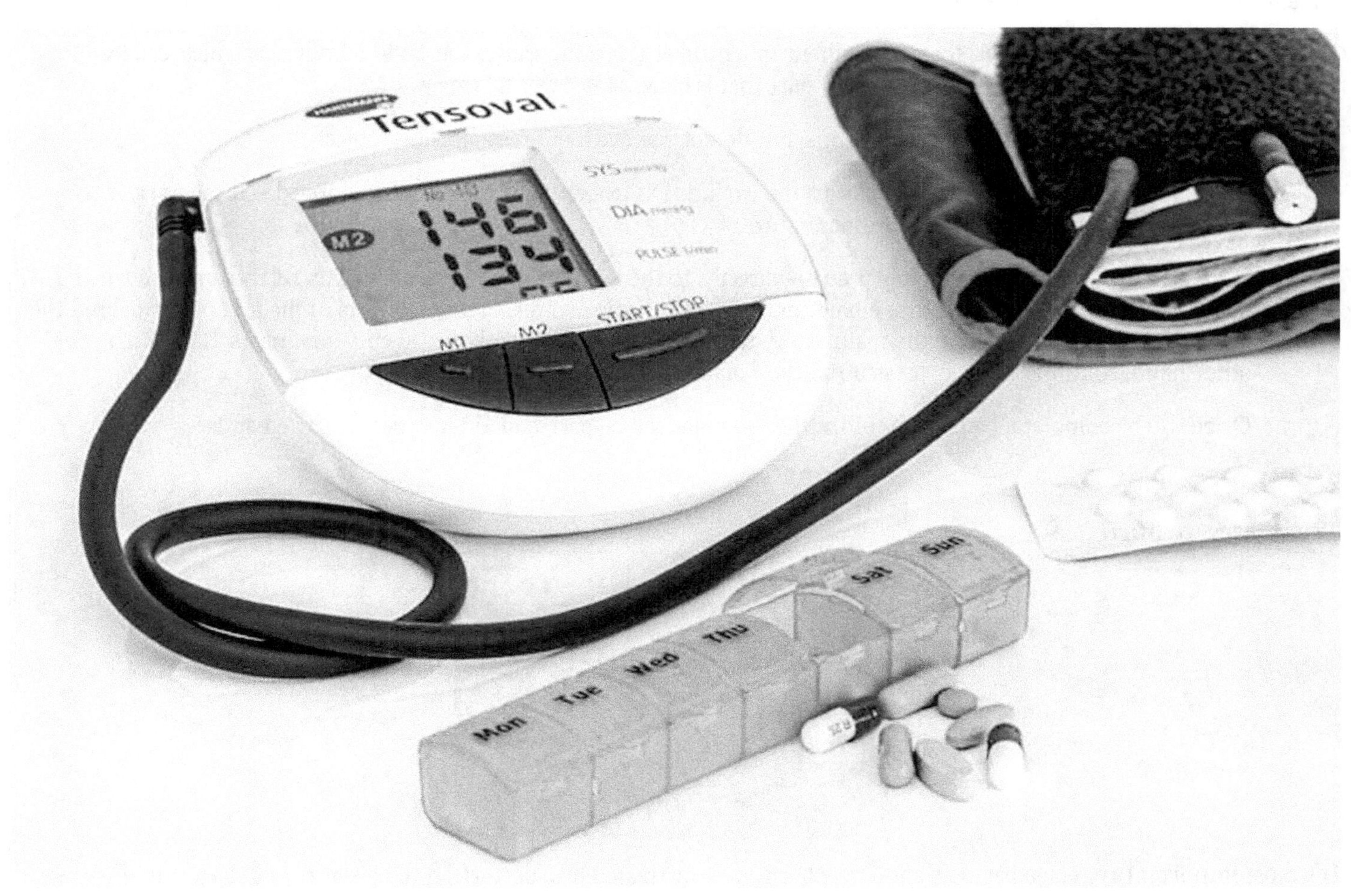

How to stop a bleeding wound

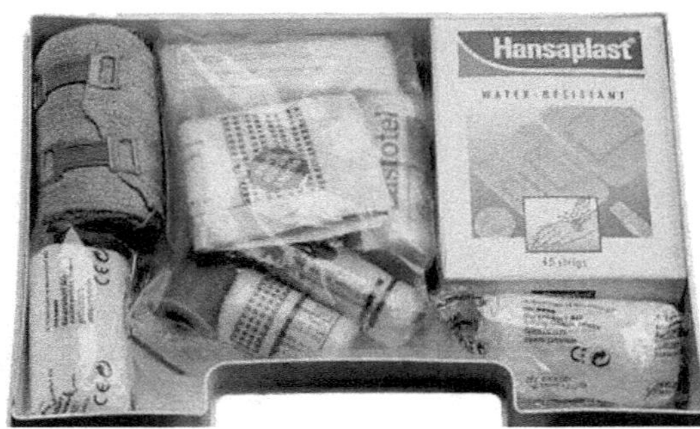

There are different kinds of bleeding, from a small open wound, to life-threatening arterial wounds. Before you start, remember to wash your hands and wear clean gloves (if you don't have a pair, a clean plastic glove will suffice.

1. Have the person lie down, then cover them in a blanket (bleeding causes you to lose body heat which can lead to hypothermia and shock), then elevate the part that is bleeding

2. Clean the wound from dirt and/or debris, but do not remove any large embedded objects.

3. Apply pressure for 20 minutes directly to the wound. Do not check if the bleeding stopped – it can cause it to restart.if there's too much blood, use more gauze.

4. If the person is still bleeding, apply pressure directly to the local artery: ""Pressure points of the arm are on the inside of the arm just above the elbow and just below the armpit. Pressure points of the leg are just behind the knee and in the groin. Squeeze the main artery in these areas against the bone. Keep your fingers flat. With your other hand, continue to exert pressure on the wound itself.

5. Once the bleeding stopped, immobilize the wounded body-part and do-not remove the bandages.

Treat a severe burn

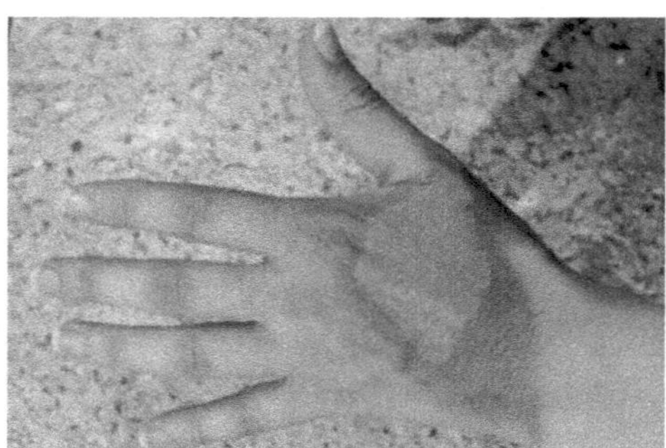

It's most important to remember that any severe burn must be treated by a doctor! In the event that a doctor is not immediately present, to treat the burn, use this method, as recommended by Dr. Matthew Hoffman:
"Immediately after a burn, run cool tap water over the skin for 10 minutes. Then, cool the skin with a moist compress. Don't put ice, butter or anything else directly on the burned skin. Clean the skin gently with mild soap and tap water. Take acetaminophen (Tylenol) or ibuprofen (Advil]) for pain. Simple burns involving only the very surface of the skin do not need dressings."

Ref: http://www.ba-bamail.com/

10 Reasons for Your Back Pain

Sudden back pain can be caused by a number of things, such as moving boxes, tough workouts, shoveling snow or carrying heavy bags. However, determining the cause of chronic back pain can be a little trickier. Let's take a look at what could potentially be to blame for your achy back.

1. **You're stressed out**
   Mental and emotional distress can manifest itself on a physiological level. If you've been feeling run down or uptight over a long period of time, muscle tension can lead to aches and spasms. Stress-triggered back pain crops up in the neck and shoulder region, as well as the lower back.
   Try: Relaxation techniques like deep breathing. Inhale slowly for a count of four, hold your breath for another count of four and exhale for a count of four. Take frequent walks and consider practicing yoga - both are also very helpful.

2. **Your heels are too high**
   While high heels may be fashionable, they could be causing you back problems. High heels throw off your center of gravity, making you lean forward when you walk. It also puts extra pressure on your feet. Consequently, this puts more stress and strain on your lower back, causing pain.
   Try: On occasions where you must wear heels (such as at the office), invest in a nice pair of walking shoes for your commute, changing your shoes when you arrive.

3. **You don't pay attention to what you eat**
   According to a 2014 study published in the Asian Spine Journal, 31 percent of women and 25 percent of men who suffered from back pain also had gastrointestinal issues, including abdominal pain and food intolerance. But what is the connection between back pain and nutrition? The main culprit here is inflammation. Foods that are high in fat and sugar cause inflammation throughout the body, including the lower back.
   Try: Cutting back on sugar and caffeine. Eat clean, whole foods instead of processed ones and always include a protein-rich food in your meals, such as meat or beans, plus whole grains such as brown rice or vegetables.

4. **Your pants are too tight**
   Outfits that are too tight constrict the body, limiting your range of motion, straining your back, neck and shoulders. Skinny jeans and pencil skirts are the worst culprits.
   Try: Opting for clothes that are snug but have a bit of a stretch to them. Make sure that you can easily slip a finger under the waistband.

5. **You sit down all day**
   One of the most detrimental things you can do to your health is sit down all day, as your muscles get used to that position, causing them to tighten up.
   Try: Reducing the effect of sitting-induced muscle stiffness and tightness by stretching your calves, hamstrings and glutes when you wake up. When these muscles begin to tighten, the lower back suffers. Also aim for a quick stretch midday and before bed. And try to get up and walk around a few times throughout the day.

6. **You smoke**
   A Northwestern University study found that smokers are three times more likely than nonsmokers to develop chronic back pain. Smoking affects how the brain responds to back pain, making people who smoke less resilient to an episode of pain. The study also found that smokers who kicked their nicotine habit during the trials experienced a decrease in chronic pain. Furthermore, previous studies found that smoking may damage tissue in the lower back area, as it slows down circulation and reduces the flow of nutrients to back muscles.

7. **You're dehydrated**
   Your spine is made up of 33 vertebrae. Between each disk is a jelly-like substance made up of 90 percent water. In order to keep that cushioning intact, your body needs a steady stream of fluid. When your body is dehydrated, those disks become flatter and less cushiony, which can consequently lead to pain.
   Try: A good way to know if you are drinking enough water is to look at the color of your urine. It should be clear or light yellow. If it is dark yellow, grab a glass of water. These tips will help you get more water in your system.

8. **You've been skipping ab workouts**

   If your abdominal muscles are weak, your lower back muscles have to work harder, which can cause lower back pain. Combat an achy back with an abdominal muscles workout. Also pay attention to how you are sitting or walking. Your core should never be relaxed - this is what often puts you at risk of developing pain.

   Try: If you're up for the challenge, there are a number of stomach crunching exercises you can try. These exercises will engage your erector spinae, the muscle that keeps your spine erect, helping you maintain correct posture. You can also try these 8 strength training exercises to slowly build up the muscles in your core before attempting a more challenging workout.

9. **Your hips are uneven**

   Many people have no idea that one side of their pelvis is slightly higher than the other. This imbalance can cause lower back pain in your day-to-day life. An apparent way to tell if your hips are uneven is during a workout, enabling you to see how your body responds to certain moves. For example, if your left hip is higher than your right when you do a lunge on the left side, you may feel that hip muscle pull tighter.

   Try: Prior to establishing a routine to cure your alignment, it is vital that you visit your doctor in order to detect any potential imbalances.

10. **You have a urinary tract infection**

    A urinary tract infection is often accompanied by pain in the lower and upper back, or sharp pains along the side. Back pain often indicates that a urinary tract infection has spread to the kidneys.

    Try: Classic UTI symptoms also include a persistent urge to urinate or pain during urination, so be sure to visit a doctor immediately for treatment.

Ref: http://www.ba-bamail.com/

When Is Chest Pain a Heart Attack?

If you wake up in the middle of the night with chest pain, your mind might automatically think you're having a heart attack. After all, it's the number one killer disease in the USA. And the number one symptom is the vague term "chest pain", which can be misleading because it's not always painful nor always in the chest. In most cases, people imagine they will have *severe* chest pain and dismiss the actual symptoms of a heart attack, go back to sleep and suffer one. Below I will discuss the symptoms you will and won't feel if you are having a heart attack and what you should do, and in which cases you should seek help immediately.

How chest pain from a heart attack feels

The typical pain described is a feeling of **tightness, squeezing or heaviness** in the chest. The Latin term *angina pectoris*, meaning sensation in the chest, is a more accurate description. This pain has been described as feeling like a band or weight is being tightened around your chest. The pain is often on the left side and above the bottom ribcage, although it's often difficult to determine its exact location.

Other typical symptoms include:

- Shortness of breath
- Sweating, nausea, and anxiety
- Pain in the left arm, jaw or neck.

What other symptoms might I feel?

While the typical symptoms are definitely a reason to visit your physician, sometimes people feel less typical pains, which could also indicate that you are having a heart attack.

- **Pain not on the left side** – sometimes the pain is located on the right, center or top of the abdomen.
- **No pain** – some people don't experience pain and only feel shortness of breath. Research indicates that no chest pain symptoms can occur in 1/3 of people having a heart attack.
- **Sharper pain** - some people report sharper chest pains or the feeling of indigestion.

How long should the chest pain last?

The next indication of whether you are suffering a heart attack is pain duration. Consider the following 3 factors:

1. Heart-attack-related chest pain comes on over several minutes and not suddenly. Sudden severe pain is a reason for concern, but it is not consistent with angina.

2. The chest pain lasts for at least 5 minutes and doesn't last continuously for more than 20 to 30 minutes.

3. Pain that comes on during rest, or doesn't go away after exertion, also indicates a heart attack.

Do I have any of the major risk factors?

Doctors like to consider the risk factors when determining whether your chest pain is a heart attack. They will take high-risk patients with atypical symptoms more seriously than low-risk patients with classic symptoms.

- **Age** – the risk increases as you age. For men it's after the age of 40 and for women it's after the age of 50. It *can* happen to a younger person, but it's more unlikely.
- **Sex** – this is not to say women aren't affected by heart disease, but the risk for heart attacks is higher for men.
- **Genetics** – your risk is significantly higher if a member of your immediate family had or has coronary heart disease. The risk is even higher if that family member was a man under 50 or a woman under 60.
- **Hypertension, diabetes, and cholesterol** – these diseases increase your risk of having a heart attack considerably.
- **Smoking** – while most people think smoking destroys your lungs (and it does), more smokers die from heart disease. Smoking substantially increases the risk of you having a heart attack.

What it shouldn't feel like

Some chest pain is not consistent with having a heart attack.

- **Sharp and brief pain** – stabbing pain that lasts only a few seconds is not coming from the heart.
- **Persists for hours** – heart attack chest pain will last for 20-30 minutes at the most and typically ends with a heart attack.
- **Gets worse with movement** – the sort of pain that worsens when pressed on is usually from chest bone or muscle pains and not the heart.
- **You can pinpoint the pain with a single finger** – heart chest pain tends to be difficult to locate exactly.

If you have a worrying pain, there is **no harm** in having it checked out. It's better to have lesser symptoms checked out than to stay at home and actually have a heart attack. **If** you are high risk, don't hesitate to have the pain checked out. **If** you are high risk and have the classical symptoms, **I** advise going to the emergency room or calling an ambulance.

H/T: www.quickanddirtytips.com

A Guide to Understanding Psoriasis

What is Psoriasis?

People with psoriasis, (pronounced suh-RY-uh-sus) have a fault in their immune system that results in an over-production of skin cells. Their bodies don't know how to get rid of these extra cells, and they cause build ups on the skin, resulting in red scaly patches. It is important to note, however, that it is not a contagious disease.

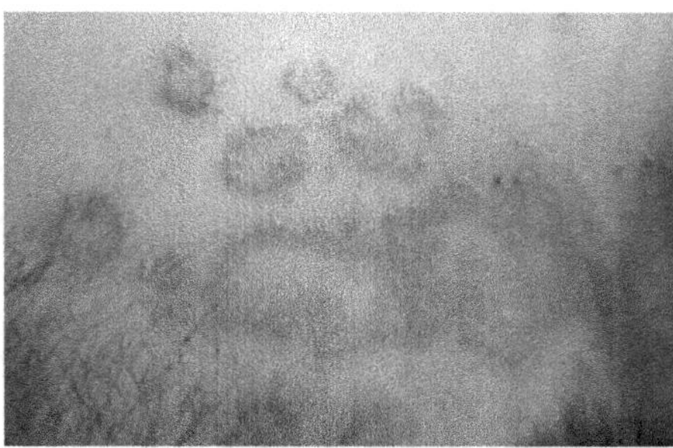

Plaque Psoriasis is the most common form and affects 90% of psoriasis patients. The skin features inflamed raised patches, usually seen on elbows, knees, the scalp and the lower back. These patches are typically covered with white or silver scales, which can itch and burn.

Guttate Psoriasis is more common in children or teenagers and is often triggered by upper respiratory infections. It features small pink to red spots and are located on the buttocks, upper arm, thighs, and scalp areas.

Psoriatic Arthritis is when you have psoriasis and then develop arthritis (inflammation of the joints). The symptoms include joint pain, stiffness and swelling of fingers and toes.

Inverse Psoriasis is seen in areas of the body with folds, usually in the armpits, groin, under the breasts, and around the genitals and buttocks. These skin regions feature smooth red plaques of skin.

Erythrodermic Psoriasis is rare and very serious. The symptoms are fiery red skin, peeling, itching, burning, an increased heart rate and changes in body temperatures. This causes protein and fluid loss, leading to infection, pneumonia, or congestive heart failure. If you have these symptoms, go to a doctor or hospital immediately.

Pustular Psoriasis mostly occurs in adults. Pustules, which are pus-filled bumps, surround red skin and form on one area of the skin. If this skin irritation is body wide, this is a more severe condition. You should seek medical attention immediately.

Treatments

Topical Medication: These are creams that can be spread over the affected areas. Usually they include steroids or vitamin B3, which aim to slow the growth of the excess skin cells. Some are available over the counter such as corticosteroid. Other well known topical medicines are calcipotriene, anthralin or tars.

Phototherapy: This is also called light therapy and employs ultraviolet light to slow down the excessive skin cell growth. Sometimes doctors use creams together with the light to treat psoriasis.

Oral Medications: Only prescribed for more severe psoriasis cases these pills or biologics work to slow the growth of skin cells. Doctors are cautious in prescribing these as they have dangerous side effects on the kidney and liver.

Things to Avoid

Cold dry climates: It is thought that cold weather worsens symptoms while hot and humid weather conditions are said to alleviate symptoms.

Scratching, picking or peeling skin: Be gentle with your skin by avoiding cuts or scrapes. Patches of psoriasis often form around injuries. Be careful when trimming your nails, as this is a common site for psoriasis to flare.

Stress and anxiety can worsen symptoms or causes flares.

Smoking and alcohol cause flares. Quit smoking and limit your daily alcohol intake.

Overexposure to sunlight: Sunburn can lead to flares of psoriasis, and of course skin damage and skin cancer. Shorter periods of sun exposure help relieve psoriasis

Some medications have been linked to aggravating psoriasis symptoms including non-steroidal anti-inflammatory drugs, beta-blockers, and lithium.

Treating Psoriasis at Home

Occlusion therapy. This therapy involves applying moisturizer to an area of skin, and then covering it with a wrap of fabric, or plastic, overnight. In the morning you should exfoliate. The occlusion keeps the skin moist and allows the medicated creams to work more effectively. It's best to discuss this method with your doctor as certain steroids and creams can have dire side effects.

Water Therapy & Dead Sea Salts: A 15-minute soak in a bath full of Dead Sea salts has been shown to soothe itchy skin and remove some of the scales. It is recommended to put a moisturizer on afterwards.
Swimming in seawater can also help as the salt in the water helps remove dead skin and scales caused by psoriasis to be loosened. It is also recommended that you shower and moisturize afterwards.

Cayenne Pepper Paste: Application of this paste to the skin reduces pain and itching. Initially you will experience a burning sensation but with subsequent applications the burning will diminish. Cayenne features capsaicin, the main ingredient in peppers, which produces heat and is often used as an ingredient in pain relief creams. It's important to be cautious when using this method as contact with other areas of your skin or eyes can be painful.

Ref: http://www.ba-bamail.com/

Prostate Cancer Risk Factors Men Should Know

According to the American National Cancer Institute, after skin cancer, prostate cancer is the most common type of cancer in men, and 1-in-7 will be diagnosed with it during their lifetime. This is quite the troubling statistic, especially since many men still don't even know where in their body the prostate is.

The prostate is a walnut-sized gland that is located under the bladder, at the base of the penis. It is a vital part of the reproductive system and its function is to assure the arrival of the sperm into the vagina. It does that by producing an alkaline fluid that protects the spermatozoa from the acidic conditions in the cervix.

While age is the number-1 risk factor when it comes to prostate cancer, there are several other key factors that can raise and lower the risks. Here are the 10 most important ones every man should know.

1. **Family History**

   If your 1st-degree relative was diagnosed with prostate cancer in the past, your risk factor is nearly double that of a person without a family history of prostate cancer. Just like how heart diseases can be hereditary, so does prostate cancer, according to a study from 2000.

2. **Excess Weight**

   Being overweight increases your risk of developing various forms of cancer, including prostate cancer. Overweight and obese men are also at risk for developing a more aggressive form of prostate cancer, according to a study from the San Diego Naval Medical Center.

3. **Frequency of Sexual Activity in Early Ages**

   A study published by the international BJU Magazine found that the more a 20-30 year-old male masturbates, the more likely he is to develop prostate cancer. Researchers believe it is caused by elevated levels of testosterone, which rises the more sexually active a young man is.

4. **Frequency of Sexual Activity in Men Over 50**

   On the other hand, the more frequently 50-year-olds engage in sexual activities, the less likely are they to develop prostate cancer, according to a study published in the Journal of Sexual Medicine. Lab tests found that the biochemical composition of sperm changes when a man engages in intercourse versus masturbation, and that change significantly affects the risk of prostate cancer. Researchers suggest that intercourse stimulates the prostate to remove toxins that masturbation does not.

5. **Frequency of Exercise**

   How much time you spend in the gym can directly affect the likeliness of you developing prostate cancer. A Harvard University study found that moderate physical exercise provides a boost to the immune system, encouraging it to produce "hunter cells" and protective chemicals that battle cancerous cells. In addition, it is speculated that burning fat also decreases prostate cancer risks.

6. **Previous Dealings with Cancer**

   Men who suffered from other forms of cancer in the past are more likely to develop prostate cancer. Studies found that men who suffered from cancer in the kidneys, bladder, lungs, thyroid and skin cancers are at a much higher risk group to develop prostate cancer.

7. **STDs**

   Suffering from infections or prostatitis can increase your chances of contracting prostate cancer. According to a University of Michigan study, men who had gonorrhea or syphilis are more likely to develop prostate cancer, especially in chronic cases. It's important to mention that these findings are still inconclusive, and another assumption is that men who suffer from STDs get checked more often, thus increasing the chances of diagnosing a preexisting condition.

8. **Alcoholism**

   Even though one glass of wine per day is good for your heart, drinking hard liquor more than 5 times a week doubles the risk of developing prostate cancer, according to a University of California study. It is still not clear how alcohol increases the risk factor, but researchers suggest that it interrupts the body's natural DNA repair mechanisms.

9. **A Calcium-Rich Diet**

   Researchers are still not sure how our eating habits affect prostate cancer risks, but several studies have found that a calcium-rich diet increases the risk of prostate cancer. Men between the ages of 19 and 70 are advised not to consume more

than 1,000mg of calcium a day, and men over 71 should limit themselves to 1,200mg per day.
It is also highly recommended not to consume more than 2,000mg per day.

10. Vasectomy

A <u>Harvard School of Public Health study</u> found that men who went through a vasectomy have a 10% increase in their risk to develop prostate cancer. In addition, the earlier in life the procedure was performed, the higher the risk. It is important to note that the American Urologist Association objects to these findings.

So What Can You Do to Minimize the Risks?

Most of the risk factors are genetic, and it is still impossible to change one's genetic makeup. However, if you maintain a healthy diet, you can significantly decrease your chances of developing prostate cancer.
It is highly advisable for men over 40 to get a checkup every year, and even more often if you're in one of the aforementioned risk groups.

Ref: http://www.ba-bamail.com/

Misleading and Far Too Common Diabetes Myths Debunked

There are many misleading myths surrounding diabetes. Unfortunately for me, I took some of these myths at face value and believed them to be true. Coming across this article really helped me to separate fact from fiction about this disease, which affects millions around the world. Here are 12 diabetes-related myths debunked:

Myth 1: Diabetes isn't a serious disease.

Fact: Diabetes IS a serious, chronic disease, however its effects can be controlled if managed properly. Nevertheless, it still kills more people annually than breast cancer and AIDS combined. Two out of three people with diabetes die from heart disease or stroke.

Myth 2: Diabetes is a death sentence.

Fact: This isn't true. The better diabetics take care of themselves, the longer they will live. Doctor's recommendations with regard to diet and exercise should be followed closely, ensuring that medication is taken correctly.

Myth 3: You'll get diabetes if you're overweight or obese.

Fact: While weight is a risk factor for diabetes, there are other factors at play too, such as family history. Many overweight people never develop Type 2 diabetes. There are also many Type 2 diabetics with a normal weight.

Myth 4: You can't do too much exercise if you have diabetes.

Fact: While it's true that diabetics who take insulin or other medications that increase insulin production in the body have to balance exercise, insulin levels and diet, those who are taking oral medications such as metformin and sitagliptin can exercise as much as they like.

Myth 5: Insulin will do you harm.

Fact: Insulin is actually a lifesaver, but what makes it challenging is that many people find it difficult to manage. Taking insulin safely requires testing blood sugar levels many times a day to avoid harmful low blood sugar reactions.

Myth 6: Diabetes means you don't produce enough insulin.

Fact: This is true for people with type 1 diabetes – their pancreas stops producing insulin completely. Those who have the more common type of diabetes, type 2, tend to have sufficient insulin when they're first diagnosed. The main problem type 2 diabetics have is that their insulin doesn't cause the cells in their bodies to absorb glucose from the food they eat. Their pancreases may also stop producing enough insulin with the passage of time, which means they'll need injections.

Myth 7: Diabetes means you have to inject yourself.

Fact: Injections are only applicable to diabetics who are on injectable medications. These days, insulin pens that don't require injections are available. Furthermore, drawing blood to measure blood sugar is painless thanks to the latest blood sugar meters. Many new diabetes medications can also be taken orally.

Myth 8: Eating too much sugar causes diabetes.

Fact: The only shred of truth in this myth is that recent research has indicated those who were already at risk of developing diabetes increased their risk of developing it further by drinking lots of sugared drinks. Sugar in itself, doesn't cause diabetes, however it does contribute to obesity, which is a major cause of the disease.

Myth 9: "I know exactly when my blood sugar is high or low."

Fact: This one is particularly dangerous, because some diabetics tend to rely on how they're feeling as a gauge for whether their blood sugar levels are low. While certain symptoms are indicative of low blood sugar levels, they tend to become less accurate over time. The only sure-fire way of knowing whether they're low or not is to actually check.

Myth 10: Diabetics cannot eat sweets.

Fact: Diabetics can eat whatever they want, as long as they pay attention to portion sizes and how often they're eating their favorite treat - what they cannot do is eat too much of what they like. An example of this is having a smaller piece of cake than usual for dessert, and not having dessert as often.

Myth 11: Diabetes makes you more prone to colds or flu.

Fact: While diabetics are no more vulnerable to contagious illnesses than anyone else, getting flu shots is important, because diabetics are a lot more likely to suffer serious complications from the flu than those who do not have the disease.

Myth 12: Diabetics on insulin haven't taken care of themselves.

Fact: During the early stages of the disease, or just after diagnosis, insulin levels can be controlled adequately through eating a healthy diet, exercising and oral medications. As the disease progresses, your pancreas may begin to produce less insulin or stop producing insulin completely, which means that you'll require insulin injections.

Ref: http://www.ba-bamail.com/

25 Things You Can Do to Prevent Alzheimer's

Alzheimer's strikes fear in all of us. The thought of losing your mind as you grow older is terrifying and made worse by the fact that, before now, there appeared to be little we could do to slow down or avoid Alzheimer's, the most common form of dementia.

Today, research has found many factors that raise or diminish the risk of Alzheimer's disease. Following these tips, you could slash your chances of developing the disease:

1. **Check out your ankle**
   Low blood flow in your foot is a clue to trouble in your brain and a simple test can reveal its cognitive state and your likelihood of stroke and dementia. The theory is that the health of your blood vessels is similar throughout the body. The degree of clogged arteries and blood flow in the feet can suggest atherosclerosis in cerebral blood vessels. Ask your doctor for an ankle-brachial index (ABI) test which involves an ultrasound device and a blood pressure cuff that compares blood pressure in your ankle with that in your arm. To remedy any impairment of blood flow your GP may advise stepped-up exercise or a change in diet/medication.

2. **Antioxidant-rich foods**
   Certain foods infuse your brain with antioxidants that can slow memory decline and help prevent Alzheimer's. All fruit and vegetables are good but top of the list are black raspberries, elderberries, raisins and blueberries.

3. **Beware of bad fats**
   The type of fat you eat changes your brain's functioning for better or worse. Stay away from saturated fats which strangle brain cells causing them to become inefficient. Buy low fat or fat-free dairy products including milk, cheese and ice cream. Cut down on deep-fried foods.

4. **Chocolate Treat**
   Cocoa, the main ingredient in chocolate, has sky-high concentrations of antioxidants called flavanols, which possess strong heart and brain-protecting properties. Drinking cocoa increases blood flow to the brain. Cocoa powder has twice as many flavanols as dark chocolate which has twice a many as milk chocolate. White chocolate has zero.

5. **Grow a bigger brain**
   Your brain starts to shrink when you reach 30 or 40 so it takes longer to learn. However scientists now believe you can increase the size of your brain through the act of learning. Try studying, learning new things or broadening your circle of friends for stimulation.

6. **The Estrogen Evidence**
   Sixty eight per cent of Alzheimer's patients are women, possibly as midway through life they lose the protection of the hormone estrogen which boosts memory. Unless your GP says otherwise, start taking estrogen immediately at the time of menopause – starting any later risks dementia and strokes.

7. **Raise good cholesterol**
   It's well known that having high good-type HDL blood cholesterol protects you from heart disease. But it can also save your brain. Researchers claim it blocks sticky stuff that destroys brain cells and acts as an anti- inflammatory to lessen brain damage. Ways to ramp up good cholesterol include exercise, drinking moderate amounts of alcohol and losing weight.

8. **Google something**
   Doing an internet search can stimulate ageing brains even more than reading a book. And MRI scans show that savvy surfers have twice as many sparks of brain activity as novices. Go online to search for information, things to buy or games to play. Although it's not known how much it will benefit your brain, it's better than passive pursuits.

9. **The ApoE4 gene**
   One in four of you reading this has a specific genetic time bomb that makes you 3 to 10 times more susceptible to developing late-onset Alzheimer's. The gene is called apolipoprotein E4. If you inherit a single variant of ApoE4 from one parent, your Alzheimer's risk triples. If you inherit a double dose from both parents, your risk rises by 10 times. Ask your doctor about a DNA test to reveal your ApoE4 genotype.

10. Say yes to coffee

Coffee is emerging as a tonic for the ageing brain. It is anti-inflammatory, helps block the ill effects of cholesterol in the brain and cuts the risks of stroke, depression and diabetes, all promoters of dementia. It is also high in antioxidants and caffeine which stop neuronal death and lessen diabetes, high blood pressure and strokes that bring on dementia. For most people, a moderate daily intake of coffee, two to four cups, won't hurt and may help.

11. Dangers of underweight

Unexplained weight loss after age 60 or so may be a sign of Alzheimer's. A study showed that women with the disease started losing weight at least 10 years before dementia was diagnosed. Among women of equal weight, those who went on to develop dementia slowly became thinner over three decades and, when diagnosed, weighed an average 12lb less that women who were free of Alzheimer's. Talk to your doctor about unexplained weight loss after 60.

12. Drink wine

A daily glass of wine may help delay dementia. Research says that alcohol is an anti-inflammatory and raises good cholesterol which helps ward off dementia. High antioxidants in red wine give it additional anti-dementia clout. Such antioxidants act as artery relaxants, dilating blood vessels and increasing blood flow which encourages cognitive functioning.

13. Know the early signs

Memory problems are not the first clue. You may notice a decline in depth perception, for example you reach to pick up a glass of water and miss it. Or you misjudge the distance in walking across a street.

Doing a jigsaw puzzle or reading a map may also be confusing. Losing your sense of smell can also be an early clue, as well as asking the same question repeatedly or misplacing belongings in odd places (like putting keys in the fridge). Be aware of memory problems as the earlier the signs are spotted, the more successful lifestyle changes and medications are likely to be.

14. A Mediterranean diet

The Mediterranean diet, no matter where you live, can help save your brain from memory deterioration and dementia. Studies consistently find that what the Greeks and Italians eat is truly brain food. Following this diet – rich in green leafy vegetables, fish, fruits, nuts, legumes, olive oil and a little vino – can cut your chances of Alzheimer's by nearly half. Rather than depending on just one food or a few nutrients, it is a rich menu of many complex brain benefactors, including an array of antioxidants, which shield brain cells from oxidative damage.

15. Middle Age Obesity

Your brain cares if you are fat. A study showed obese people had 8% less brain tissue and overweight people had 4% less brain tissue than people of average weight, which according to some scientists hugely increases the risk of Alzheimer's. Moreover, brain shrinkage occurred in areas of the brain targeted by Alzheimer's, and which are critical for planning, long-term memory, attention and executive functions, and control of movement.

Tackle signs of rising weight early, when you are young or middle-aged. Oddly, being obese after the age of 70 does not raise the risk of Alzheimer's but that doesn't mean you should neglect exercise as it is the best way of stimulating cognitive functioning and may delay the onset of Alzheimer's at any age.

16. Get a good night's sleep

A lack of sleep is toxic to brain cells. Sleep has surprising powers to protect your brain against memory loss and Alzheimer's. It is a wonder drug that helps manipulate levels of the dreaded brain toxin peptide beta-amyloid, a prime instigator of Alzheimer's, which according to one scientist puts you at accelerated risk. Research has also found that sleeping an average of five hours or less a night is linked to large increases in dangerous visceral abdominal fat, which can cause diabetes and obesity that can lead to Alzheimer's. Take naps and seek treatment for sleep disorders.

17. Have an extended social circle

Studying the brain of a highly sociable 90-year-old woman who died from Alzheimer's, researchers in Chicago found that having a large social network provided her with strong "cognitive reserve" that enabled her brain to not realize she had Alzheimer's. Why this happens is a mystery but interacting with friends and family seems to make the brain more efficient. It finds alternative routes of communication to bypass broken connections left by Alzheimer's. So see friends and family often and expand your social network. The stronger the brain reserve you build through life, the more likely you are to stave off Alzheimer's symptoms.

18. Deal with stress

When you are under stress, your body pours out hormones called corticosteroids, which can save you in a crisis. But persistent stress reactions triggered by everyday events like work frustration, traffic and financial worries can be dangerous. Over time, it can destroy brain cells and suppress the growth of new ones, actually shrinking your brain. Sudden traumatic events like the death of a loved one or a life-changing event like retirement can leave a hangover of severe psychological stress that precedes dementia. Be aware that chronic stress can increase older people's vulnerability to memory decline and dementia. Seek professional advice. Antidepressants, counselling, relaxation techniques and other forms of therapy may head off stress-related memory loss if treated early.

19. Take care of your teeth

Bad gums may poison your brain. People with tooth and gum disease tend to score lower in memory and cognition tests, according to US dental researchers who found that infection responsible for gum disease gives off inflammatory byproducts that travel to areas of the brain involved in memory loss. Consequently, brushing, flossing and preventing gum disease may help keep your gums and teeth healthy but also your memory sharper. In another study, older people with the most severe gingivitis — inflamed gums — were two to three times more likely to show signs of impaired memory and cognition than those with the least.

20. Get enough Vitamin B12

As you age, blood levels of vitamin B12 go down and the chance of Alzheimer's goes up. Your ability to absorb it from foods diminishes in middle age, setting the stage for brain degeneration years later. Researchers at Oxford University found that a brain running low on B12 actually shrinks and a shortage can lead to brain atrophy by ripping away, myelin, a fatty protective sheath around neurons. It can also trigger inflammation, another destroyer of brain cells. Take 500 to 1000mcg of vitamin B12 daily after the age of 40. If you or an older family member has unexplained memory loss, fatigue or signs of dementia, be sure to get tested for vitamin B12 deficiency by your GP.

21. Vinegar in everything

There is plenty of evidence that vinegar sinks risk factors that may lead to memory decline, namely high blood sugar, insulin resistance, diabetes and pre-diabetes and weight gain. Researchers in Phoenix, Arizona, have noted in studies of humans and animals that the acidic stuff packs potent glucose-lowering effects. Studies have also found it can curb appetite and food intake, helping prevent weight gain and obesity, which are associated with diabetes, accelerated dementia and memory loss. Pour on the vinegar — add it to salad dressings, eat it by the spoonful, even mix it into a glass of drinking water. Any type of vinegar works.

22. Have your eyes checked

If you preserve good or excellent vision as you age, your chances of developing dementia drop by an astonishing 63%. And if it's poor, just visiting an optician for an eye test and possible treatment at least once in later life cuts your dementia odds by about the same amount. Exactly how vision problems promote dementia is not clear but impaired vision makes it difficult to participate in mental and physical activities such as reading and exercising, as well as social activities, all believed to delay cognitive decline. Be aware that your eyes reflect and influence how your brain is functioning, especially as you age. Don't tolerate poor vision as often it can be corrected.

23. Eat curry or take curcumin pills

Curry powder contains the yellow-orange spice turmeric, packed with curcumin, a component reported to stall memory decline. One study showed elderly Indians who ate even modest amounts of curry did better in cognitive tests. Curcumin works by blocking the build-up of Alzheimer's-inducing amyloid plaques (deposits found in the brains of sufferers) then nibbles away at existing plaques to slow cognitive decline.

It is recommended to eat two or three curries a week, and make it a yellow curry. Otherwise, sprinkle the spices on your food. Read more about the many benefits of Curcumin.

24. diabetes control

Having type 2 diabetes makes you more vulnerable to Alzheimer's. Studies show it may double or triple your risk and the earlier diabetes takes hold, the higher the odds of dementia. Some experts refer to Alzheimer's as "diabetes of the brain". The two disorders have similar causes — obesity, high blood pressure, high cholesterol, high fat and high sugar diets, low physical activity as well as high blood sugar. In short, diabetes can deliver a double whammy to the brain, destroying neurons and increasing inflammation. Do everything possible to keep blood sugar levels low and stick to a low-saturated-fat diet and regular exercise.

25. Drink more tea

Evidence suggests that tea stalls the cognitive loss that precedes Alzheimer's and that the more tea you drink, the sharper your ageing memory is. Tea's secret is no mystery. The leaves are packed with compounds able to penetrate the blood-brain barrier and block neuronal damage.

One particular green tea antioxidant can block the toxicity of beta-amyloid, which kills brain cells. Make a point of drinking black and green tea. Don't add milk, it can reduce tea's antioxidant activity by 25%.

Ref: http://www.ba-bamail.com/

Prevent Alzheimer's with a Healthy Lifestyle

While the medical world has urgently been seeking to cure Alzheimer's disease with pharmaceuticals, studies in this field have discovered that prevention is also worth exploring. Researchers have found that everyday behaviors, which unlike genetics are within our control, can boost brain reserves and therefore help delay or even prevent the onset of Alzheimer's or dementia.

1. **Exercise regularly**

   Research reveals that your risk of developing Alzheimer's disease can be reduced by 50% with regular exercise. Exercise also helps slow down deterioration when you have already begun developing cognitive problems.
   Start small. Exercise can be overwhelming for those who don't do it regularly. You can start by taking the stairs or walking when you are talking on your cell phone.
   30 minutes, 5 times a week. This seems like a lot, but it can include activities that get your heart pumping, such as cleaning, gardening or doing laundry. You can also walk, try an aerobics class, or swim.
   Protect your head. Trauma to the head increases your chances of developing cognitive issues. Sports such as football and boxing are more extreme examples, but even a fall from a bicycle can have an effect. Wear the correct headgear and fasten your seat belt in cars.
   Balance and coordination. Similarly, you can help prevent future head injuries caused by falling by including exercises that help you focus on balance and coordination. Yoga, Tai Chi or any exercise using balance balls or discs can help keep you agile.

2. **Be well-rested**

   Restful sleep on a regular basis helps your brain work best. Deep sleep is necessary for memory formation and retention. Sleep deprivation slows your thinking and has been shown to increase the chances of Alzheimer's disease symptoms.
   Regular sleep schedule: Our brain's clock responds well to regularity. Make sure to go to sleep and wake up at a similar time each day to correspond to our natural circadian rhythms.
   Smart napping: Napping can interfere with your regular sleep and make your insomnia worse. If you do nap, make sure it's for no more than 30 minutes and do so in the early afternoon.
   Bedroom sanctity: Ban computers and televisions from the bedroom as these stimulators distract you from sleep.
   Relaxing bedtime routine: Having pre-bedtime activities such as having a bath, light stretching, dimming the lights, praying or writing in a journal help signify to your brain that it's time for restorative sleep.

3. **Keep mentally stimulated**

   People who are mentally active have been found to be more protected against developing Alzheimer's and dementia. Any activities requiring communicating, interacting or organizing have proven tremendously helpful.
   Learn a new skill. Learning a new skill helps make larger deposits in the brain reserves. Try studying a new language, learn to play an instrument, read the paper or books, or take up a new hobby.
   Memory exercises: Memorization builds your memory connections. Start with memorizing something small like capital cities or a poem, then progress to rhymes and mnemonics.
   Brain games: Try riddles, crossword puzzles or strategy games. Play board or card games, word games like Scrabble or Boggle, or number puzzles like Sudoku. All of these help build your capacity to retain cognitive associations.
   The 5 Ws: Keep your neurons firing by asking yourself "Who, what, where, when and why?". Follow this up by writing down your daily experiences.
   Go off routine: Varying habits helps create new brain pathways. Take a new route, use your non-dominant hand, or rearrange a storage system in your home.

4. **Eat healthily**

   A nutritious diet optimizes your brain's performance. Changes to your diet can help keep you protected against brain deterioration.

Skip trans-fats and saturated fats. Choose lean meats, less processed foods, skim or fat-free dairy products, and reduce your intake of fried foods.

Adopt a Mediterranean diet. This diet, consisting of fish, nuts, whole grains, olive oil, fresh fruit and vegetables, with the occasional glass of wine or piece of dark chocolate, is good for your heart. A healthy heart helps lower the risk of developing Alzheimer's disease.

Eat fish and avocado. Both are filled with omega 3, a good fatty acid, which researchers have discovered may help prevent Alzheimer's disease and dementia.

Opt for 4-6 small meals. Eating more regularly helps maintain a consistent blood sugar level.

Think rainbow: Eat an abundance of colorful fruits and vegetables to achieve a diet high in antioxidants and vitamins. Reduce the white shades of your diet too: Carbohydrates high in sugar or refined flour lead to higher glucose levels which can inflame your brain.

Drink tea: Green tea has been shown to be excellent for a focused memory and mental alertness which can slow the aging of the brain.

Ref: http://www.ba-bamail.com/

Bone Spurs: What They are and How to Treat Them

Having problems with your back can be quite a nuisance, as well as being costly to get them checked and treated. Rightly so, many back problems that are associated with bone health are very often hard to ignore seeing as the spine is such a fundamental part of our body. In addition, conditions such as arthritis can lead to further complications that might remain undetected. An example of such a complication is bone spurs.

Bone spurs (also known as osteophytes) arise as a result of excess pressure on your joints and develop as an "extra bone" produced by the body in response to this pressure. Apart from your spine, they can appear in other body parts, such as the knees, hips, shoulders, and fingers. Although their symptoms are not always obvious, they can sometimes cause pain and loss of motion in the joints. They can be treated if seen by a doctor, unless a specific case does not require treatment at all. Let's take a closer look at the symptoms, causes, treatments, and prevention of this condition.

First of all, what is a bone spur and how does it form?

A bone spur is an extra bone that forms in areas of the body where bones meet each other, such as in your joints and in your spine. When these areas experience unusual amounts of pressure and tension, the body naturally reacts by forming bone spurs in order to reduce the excess pressure. Unfortunately this isn't always helpful, and in some cases, spurs can make the situation even worst.

Weight-bearing joints, such as the knees, heels and shoulders, are the most sensitive to the formation of bone spurs, although they may also appear in the spine, hips, hands, and ankles. The risk of this sensitivity increases in people who are overweight (as this puts excess weight on the joints), in athletes (as they use a lot of force in their legs and feet when running), and in people who lift heavy objects on a regular basis (causing spurs in the shoulders).

Above all, there are major causes that depend on the presence of other bone conditions. Two of the most common ones are a degenerative joint disease (such as arthritis) and the inflexibility of a tendon. In both of these cases, the body attempts to reinforce the weak area with more bone in a place that it shouldn't be, resulting in bone spurs. These become very painful when there's no more room for the bone to grow, so it pokes into the surroundingtissue, or pulls a tendon too tightly to accommodate it.

What are the symptoms?

As a result of the contact of bone spurs with the tissue that surrounds them, the body may suffer from irritation and inflammation in the affected areas. It may appear as swelling and is felt as a sharp ache and pain. Here's how symptoms arise in specific areas:

Knees: Difficulty extending or bending your legs

Spine: Weakness or numbness in the arms and/or legs (due to the spinal cord or nerve roots being pinched) **Hip:** Reduction in the range of motion in your hip joints - this may even be felt as pain in the knees **Shoulder:** Swelling and tearing in the rotator cuff

Fingers: Appearance of hard lumps under the skin

If you experience one or more of the above symptoms, or have difficulty moving one or more joints around your body, make an appointment with your doctor, so he can detect the problem as soon as possible. Your doctor is likely to feel the bone spurs externally, or he may recommend getting an X-ray if he feels he needs to investigate further. Early treatment helps to prevent further joint damage.

How can they be treated?

Your doctor may recommend over-the-counter pain relievers or anti-inflammatory drugs if your bone spurs are causing pain or inflammation, but there are also other widely-known remedies that treat the problem. Some individuals find applying moist heat, cold packs, or ice massages to be soothing. Others suggest the use of herbs, especially chamomile, which has anti-inflammatory and pain-relieving properties. Some drug therapies, modalities, stretches, and injections may also work, always if advised by a doctor. If symptoms persist or worsen, a surgical procedure might be necessary to remove the extra bone, lengthen the affected tendon, or replace a joint. Generally, the main focus of the cure should be to tackle underlying bone problems, such as degenerative disease or tendon contracture and inflexibility. If this is not done, the bone spur might re-develop even if it was surgically removed.

How can bone spurs be prevented?

To reduce the risk of their development, you should try engaging in a stretching and/**or** weight reduction program, as well as a low-impact maintenance exercise program to strengthen your core and stretch sensitive tendons, including

your calves, hamstrings, and quads. Try walking (in supportive shoes), swimming, doing yoga, cycling, or doing any form of exercise that is a great way of keeping fit without creating pressure on the joints and tendons.

Ref: http://www.ba-bamail.com/

How to Tell If You Have a Magnesium Deficiency

Magnesium is one of those vital vitamins your body needs to work properly. Without it your body cannot effectively regulate cholesterol levels or break down fat. Magnesium also controls the production of antioxidants, proteins and enzymes. Magnesium is also responsible for creating and repairing DNA and RNA strains. Usually you get it from foods and beverages you consume, but increasingly people are suffering from deficiencies of it – four out of five Americans are said to have a deficiency. The good news is that your body lets you know when it's lacking in minerals. Here are the 8 outward warning signs that you might have a deficiency.

1. Easily injured

Magnesium plays a vital role in your muscle health and ensures that your bones and musculoskeletal system functions correctly. One consequence of a magnesium deficiency is that you develop osteoporosis. This means you will get injured fairly easily and your muscles will be much weaker, because magnesium builds blocks of muscles and produces proteins. This symptom is one of the more tell-tale ones in having a magnesium deficiency. It's recommended that you take calcium and magnesium supplements in this case.

2. Bad headaches

There are many causes behind the classic headaches but if you find yourself suffering from severe migraines or tension headaches, this could indicate a magnesium headache. You can try alter this by eating foods rich in magnesium or magnesium supplements to see if the headaches subside. If your headaches persist you should be in contact with your physician to investigate other possible causes.

3. Insomnia

While the most common cause behind the tens of millions of insomnia cases is stress, it can also be caused by a magnesium deficiency. If you find yourself having difficulty falling asleep or your waking up during the night, it's best to have your magnesium levels checked out.

4. Muscle cramps

Magnesium plays a key role in making sure your muscles are relaxed and support your body's general cellular function. Since you use your muscles daily it's important to provide them with the right minerals so that they function correctly. Both a lack of magnesium and potassium are well known causes of muscle cramps so it's recommended that you increase both of these minerals via supplements.

5. Hypertension

The leading cause behind hypertension, also called high blood pressure, is an intake in sodium. The second cause is a magnesium deficiency, and it is a notable symptom of this deficiency. It might be worth considering a magnesium supplement before resorting to strong prescription medication.

6. Anxiety and depression

A lack of magnesium might actually be bringing you down or giving you anxiety and panic attacks. Magnesium controls your mood and works to calm your body. The common modern day problems of anxiety and depression might be driven by low magnesium levels. It's worth trying magnesium supplements for a few days to see if there's a change in your mood before committing to antidepressants.

7. **Muscle pain**

Low levels of magnesium are known for causing muscle cramps it can also trigger more severe muscle pain, known as fibromyalgia. This painful symptom is a tell-tale sign of a magnesium deficiency. To test whether your fibromyalgia is magnesium related take supplement pills for a few days to see if the pain subsides.

8. **Spikes in blood sugar**

Magnesium is also an important component in leveling out your blood sugar level and works to improve glucose absorption. If you notice that your blood sugar spikes or that you are feeling tired all the time, no matter how much you eat, you might be magnesium-deficient. Similarly you might be running low on magnesium if you are chronically fatigued and develop adrenal fatigue

Ref: http://www.ba-bamail.com/

Identify & Treat Excessive Ear Wax at Home

It is easy to view ear wax as an annoyance, but like most secretions, it has an important purpose. It's a cleaning agent, produced by your ears to prevent them from drying out. It contains protective and anti- bacterial agents to help your ears stay healthy. However, various factors can cause more wax than is needed to collect in the outer part of the ear canal and if it's left unattended, it can cause pain and eventually require medical intervention. But don't worry, help is at hand in the form of these effective remedies you can try at home!

What is Ear Wax?

'Wax' is something of a misnomer for the body fluid that forms in your ear. It is actually a water-soluble mixture of various secretions mixed with hair and dead skin, formed in the outer part of the ear rather than the inner drum. Your ears are self-cleaning for the most part, and the secretions help move dead skin to the opening of the ear, aided by the jaw motion you use when you chew. Once out in the open, 'wax' will usually dry out and flake away naturally. However over time it can build up and cause other problems, sometimes aided by overproduction or a blockage within the ear canal.

What You Shouldn't Do

Firstly, don't fall into the trap of thinking that digging every last bit of wax out of your ear constantly is an indicator of good personal hygiene. Remember that ear wax has its uses and removing it excessively can cause your ear canal to dry out. However, if it accumulates in excess, it can cause discomfort and even pain. It is in these circumstances that you need to take action.
The other big 'NO' is the use of homemade poking and scraping devices down your ear hole. Q-Tips, bobby pins, pencils and any other similar instruments are NOT suitable for cleaning your ears, no matter how many times you might have used them in the past. Although you may see remnants of wax on your Q-Tip after you have had a good rummage down your ear, you will more than likely have pushed other clumps further into your ear canal. Additionally, if you prod down too far then you could cause serious damage to the inner ear.

Signs You Need to Take Action

Since you don't need to constantly clean the wax out of your ears, what are the signs that you have an excessive buildup that you need to deal with? Different ears produce different amounts of wax. It may be that you know from past experience that you are likely to have excess wax. There are a number of other signs that can indicate a problem too:

- Earache
- Strangely muffled hearing
- Tinnitus or ringing noises in ear
- Itchy ears
- Odor and noticeable, moist discharge
- An uncomfortable sensation of 'fullness' in the ear

You can buy ear drops and wax removal kits or visit your doctor, but the answer to your problems can also be found in natural remedies you can make in your own home. Here are some that have proved useful to others:
N.B. - Please note that these remedies should not be used if you have an ear infection, hearing loss or severe earache.

1. **Salt Water**
   Salt water is one of the best home remedies for excessive ear wax. It works by softening the wax inside the ear and flushing it out to the surface:

   - Take a teaspoon of salt and drop it in a half cup of warm water. Wait until the salt dissolves entirely.
   - Take a soft, cotton ball and dip it in the solution.
   - Tilt your head so that your affected ear is facing skywards. Place the cotton ball over the opening and let the solution drip into your ear canal.
   - Keep your head tilted for three to four minutes.
   - Tilt your head downwards to let any excess solution drain back out.
   - Wipe the area around the opening of your ear with a clean cloth to remove softened wax.

2. **Olive Oil**

   Olive oil can also soften ear wax. It also lists 'antiseptic properties' among its many benefits so it can help reduce your risk of an ear infection as well:

   - Slightly warm some olive oil. Make sure it isn't too hot to touch of course as you should be able to easily bear it against your skin.
   - Put two to three small drops of the oil into the ear, using a dropper or, ask someone to do it for you.
   - Let the solution settle for ten minutes and then tilt your head to remove any excess.
   - Repeat the process before bedtime for 3-4 days.

3. **Hydrogen Peroxide**

   Hydrogen peroxide is used in many of the over-the-counter ear drops you can buy for wax removal. It is important that you don't use this one if you have sensitive skin. Always make sure that the peroxide you use is less than 3% in strength:

   - Mix together equal parts water and (3% or less) hydrogen peroxide.
   - Tilt your head sideways and drop a few drops of the solution in to your ear (ask someone else to do this for you if you don't have a dropper).
   - Make sure you place a towel over your shoulder to catch any loose drips.
   - Allow the solution to stay in the ear for 10 to 15 minutes. Lie down on a pillow, keeping the treated ear pointed skywards if it helps.
   - You should feel tickling or a bubbling sensation.
   - When this sensation stops, remove the solution by tilting your head the other way, and dry your ear with a clean cloth.

4. **Vinegar and Rubbing Alcohol Solution**

   This is a remedy from a bygone age and works by dissolving the ear wax. The antibacterial properties of the vinegar also helps keep infection at bay.

   - Mix equal parts white vinegar and rubbing alcohol in a small bowl.
   - Immerse a cotton ball in the solution, then remove it.
   - Tilt your head so that the ear you want to treat is facing upwards.
   - Use the cotton ball to apply a small amount of the solution into the opening of the ear.
   - After four to five minutes, tilt your head back the other way and use a cloth to catch the liquid as it is dispelled from the ear.
   - Dab clean with a cloth or tissue.

5. **Baby Oil or Glycerin (Mineral Oil)**

   If you have either of these products lying around your house, they are great for softening up your excessive ear wax as well:

   - Use a dropper or the help of friends and family to put three drops of oil into your ear while it is facing upwards.
   - Place a cotton ball over the ear opening to help the oil stay in your ear.
   - After around ten minutes, remove the cotton ball and allow the oil to drain onto a cloth or tissue.
   - Wipe away any excess soft wax.

What To Do If Your Problems Persist

If your ear continues to feel uncomfortable after the application of these natural remedies and/or over-the- counter solutions available from the pharmacy, you will need to book an appointment with your doctor or an Ear, Nose and Throat Consultant. You should always consult a medic if you have severe ear ache, large amounts of fluid flowing, severe hearing loss, dizziness, fever and vomiting. Your ears are important, please look after them!

Ref: http://www.ba-bamail.com/

Factors that Influence Our blood sugar Levels

A big rise in blood sugar levels is an issue for everyone. Of course, this is most important to those who suffer from diabetes or have any risk factors associated with the disease.

Besides the sweets and sugar-filled desserts we all think about when we think of sugar, there are some surprising factors and other foods that can, especially over time, prevent the body from balancing its blood sugar levels. This post will explain the foods and habits you should avoid, as well as those which actually help the balance.

Sugar-free Products

Surprisingly enough and completley unfair, sugar-free foods can cause a spike in our blood sugar levels. A lot of these foods contains carbs, starch, and fat. Carbs alone are known to spike the blood sugar levels, what can cause organ damage for those suffering from diabetes.

Chinese Food

Fat-rich foods can keep the blood sugar levels higher for a longer period of time. Chinese food (especially in fast-food restaurants) contains a lot of oil as well as sugar, and so is probably not a good combination if you're diabetic or want a lower blood sugar level. This isn't to say that common oil foods like fries or pizza are a good idea either.

The Flu

Yes, unfortunately, there are situations outside our control that can spike our blood sugar levels. The extreme loss of fluids that happens during a flu attack creates a spike in the blood sugar levels. But that's not all, medicine such as antibiotics can also change the sugar balance in the body, as well as the body's actual war against the disease. That is why you should drink more and eat even less sugar and carbs during this time.

Mental Stress

Stress, from whatever source (work, personal life), can cause the body to release "stress hormones", which usually elevate the amount of sugar in the blood. Relaxation techniques such as deep breathing and meditation can alleviate the tension and reduce the sugar levels back to their proper levels.

Buns

Yes, buns. How are they different to regular bread? Well, buns usually have a better taste than regular bread, and that's because they contain quite a bit more sugar. It's better to stick to full wheat bread.

Energy Drinks

Sports drinks were initially made to allow the body to absorb liquid easily and quickly after a physical workout. But two things are important to know about them: First, they are full of sugar, and second, they are not made for the average person. They are made for athletes and runners.

Dry Fruit

Eating fruit is a very healthy choice, but not in all forms. In the case of lowering your blood sugar levels, dry fruit isn't recommended as they contain a lot of sugar for their weight. A handful of dry fruit is enough to spike your blood sugar levels.

Steroids

Allergies, as well as asthma, osteporosis, rash and many other medical problems are treated with steroids. However, you should be aware that certain types of steroids may encourage the onset of diabetes. It doesn't mean you shouldn't fill the doctor's prescription, but pointing out this fact to them and mentioning that you are at risk of diabetes can't hurt.

Factors aiding the balance of blood sugar levels

To keep a balanced level of sugar in our blood, here are a couple of tricks that can help:

Continuous mild physical activity

We're not talking about daily trips to the gym, but even daily tasks such as cleaning the house or working in the garden. This kind of ongoing activity has an excellent influence on the blood sugar levels and can significantly reduce them.

Yogurt

Yogurt contains pro-biotic agents, meaning bacteria that help our digestion. The aid to our digestive system ultimately leads to a reduction of the sugar levels in our bloodstream. Warning: One can destroy this benefit by mixing sweet or fruit-flavored yogurts.

A Vegetarian Diet

Studies have found that people who gave up meat, dairy products and eggs have had better control over

their blood sugar levels, and needed less insulin. One of the theories about this effect is that plant food, high in fiber, can slow the deconstruction of carbs and so brings about a slower, more controlled absorption of the sugar into the blood, instead of spiking it.

Cinnamon

Other than the fact that cinnamon has been, for years now, considered a home remedy that lowers the risk of diabetes, recent studies have confirmed this. Cinnamon contains natural chemicals that improve the

function of insulin and help maintain a reasonable level of sugar in the blood. In order to enjoy these advantages, add a little to every meal.

A few important notes:

- Studies have found that birth control pills can affect the blood sugar levels.

- Those who suffer from type 1 diabetes may experience a drop during the night and should consider having a little snack before, or even during, bed time.

- High-intensity physical training can cause a 'roller coaster' of blood sugar levels, meaning a spike and then a quick drop. It's important to record your blood sugar levels before, during and after a workout.

- Drinking alcoholic drinks can have the same 'roller coaster' effect. You should eat something when you drink.

- Heat can also play a role in spikes and drops in blood sugar levels. It's best to stay in cool places during hot hours, and of course - drink a lot of water.

Ref: http://www.ba-bamail.com/

Home/Natural Remedies

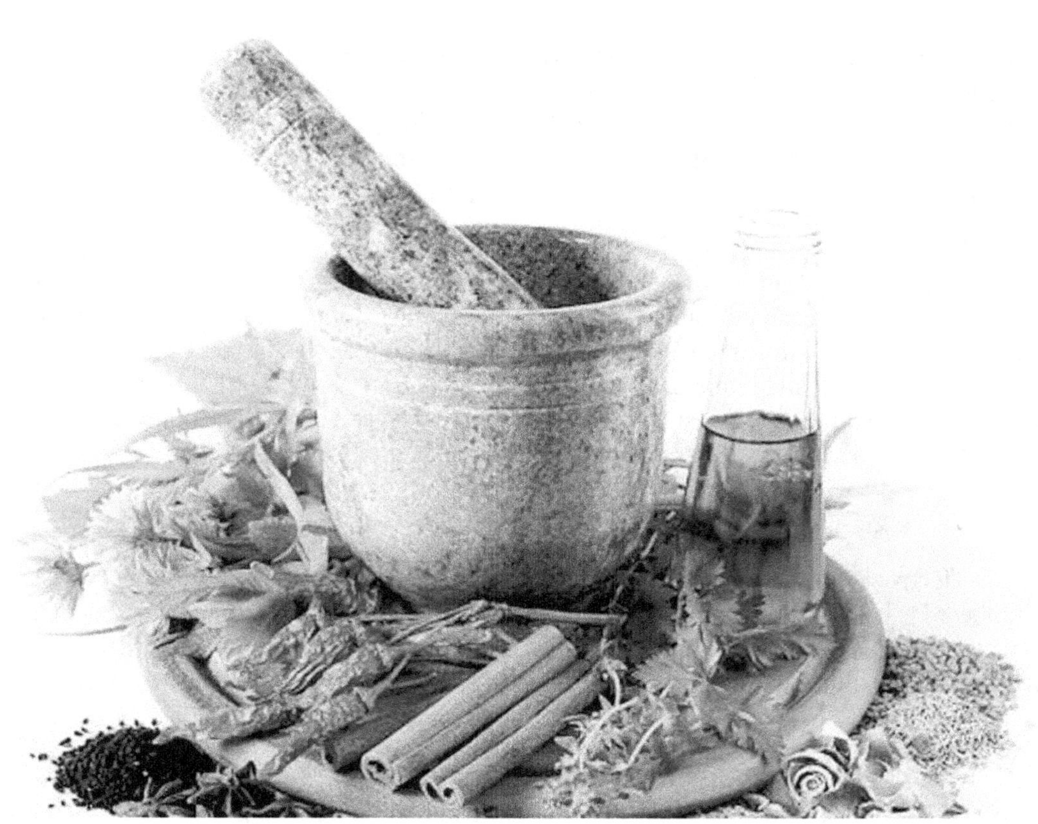

Natural healing from the Sunnah

Ibn al-Qayyim, the noted Muslim scholar stated that the principles of sound health are three:

- preservation of good health

- removal of harmful substances from the body and

- keeping the body away from harm.

In a modern context this equates to eating wholesome nutritious foods, ensuring balance of quality and quantity, keeping away from things that are toxic and harmful to the body (and in modern society there are many), and striving to detoxify the body from the consequences of bad diet and lifestyle and exposure to harmful elements.

This article will examine aspects of natural healing from the Sunnah of the Prophet Muhammad (peace be upon him).

Black Seed (Habba-tu Sawda) – Black cumin, fennel flower Abu Huraira (may Allah be pleased with him), narrated that Allah's Messenger (peace be upon him) said: "Use this black seed regularly, because it has a cure for every disease except death." (Reported by Bukhari.).

The Black seed is the common fennel flower plant (Nigella sativa) of the buttercup family. This herb grows to about 16-24 inches and has finely divided foliage with blue flowers. From this plant, comes a small black seed, which is also known as the blessed seed or black seed, and some call it the Arabian seed because of its habitat. The Black Seed plant is also known by other names, and they vary between places. The Black Seed has been used for over two thousand years. It has been said that the Black Seed should be used regularly because it has a cure for every disease except death.

A special oil is extracted from the seed which is used in the preparation of various medical formulas. It has been used to treat bronchitis and coughs. Also it has been used to help increase body tone, as a digestive tonic, to quell belching, stimulates excretion of urine, dissolves wind, quells colic pain and stomach-gas colic, expels worms, benefits some skin allergies, stimulates menstrual period, and increases the flow of breast milk. If you add a few drops to coffee or tea it can help calm the nervous system, help pertussis, dry cough, asthma, and bronchial respiratory complaints. If you take the Black Seed oil unmixed or undiluted it can produce gripe, and irritate the digestive system. The Black Seed acts as an expectorant by stimulating the body's energy and helping it to recover from fatigue and dispirtedness. (Medicine of the Prophet)

SIDE EFFECTS

Black seed is a safe and effective herb that can be used by almost anyone. No irritations or side effects are caused when the right dose is correctly applied. Its benefits are obtained through consistent use, the effects are medium to long term. Black seed can be used in the treatment of diabetes mellitus or diabetes caused by an allergy, but it is recommended that the treatment be supervised because Black seed lowers blood sugar levels. Black seed should not be taken by pregnant women.

NUTRITIONAL COMPONENTS

Black seed contains over 100 valuable nutrients. It is comprised of approximately 21% protein, 38% carbohydrates, and 35% plant fats and oils. The active ingredients of black seed are nigellone, thymoquinone, and fixed oils. Black seed also contains significant proportions of protein, carbohydrates and essential fatty acids. Other ingredients include linoleic acid, oleic acid, calcium, potassium, iron, zinc, magnesium, selenium, vitamin A, vitamin B, vitamin B2, niacin, and vitamin C. The black seed is known in Arabic as the habbutual barakah (the seed of blessing).

Dates

Dates were the food that Allah provided for Mary after she gave birth to Prophet Jesus under the palm tree. Allah inspired Jesus, her blessed infant, and his future messenger to the children of Israel, in one of the early miracles of his birth to say to her: "Shake the trunk of the palm-tree, and it will drop ripe dates on you, so eat, drink, and comfort your eyes (with what Allah gave you) (Qur'an 19:25).

Abdullaah bin Ja'afar reported that he saw Prophet Muhammad (peace be upon him) eating fresh ripe dates with cucumber (Bukhari and Muslim). Sometimes he also ate a couple of fresh dates with a drink to sweeten it. He also used to eat a couple of fresh dates for his morning breakfast and before attending fajr prayers. When he did not find fresh dates he ate dried ones.

Fresh dates stimulate sexual desire, increases semen, balances the constitution of people with cold temperament, and in general is extremely healthy and rich in benefits for the body, particularly where it is the staple fruit of the land. For those who are not used to eating it, fresh dates will break down and putrefy rapidly in the stomach, and they will generate excessive heat and boiling of the blood, causing extreme headache and imbalance of the black bile, and damaging the teeth, hence requiring balancing and adjustment of the humors through either food of cold temperament or through purgation. (Medicine of the Prophet).

It is also reported that Allah's Messenger (peace be upon him) sometimes ate dates with butter, bread, or alone. Dried dates are moist in the first degree. Many of the benefits of eating dates are prominent for the dwellers of hot climates. As for the dwellers of cold climates, particularly those who are not used to it, eating dates immoderately can cause glaring of the eyes, headache, and damage teeth. These adverse effects can be overcome by eating almonds and poppies. (Medicine of the Prophet).

Honey

"honey, in it there is a cure for people." – Qur'an 16:69,

Hot Lemon and Honey

Take the juice of a lemon and squeeze a few tablespoons into a cup. Add a tablespoon of raw, pure honey. Then cover with boiling water. Stir it and then sip it. There is a cure in honey and lemon is a cleanser and a purifier. This mixture is great for sore throats, colds, or just as a general pick me up. Enjoy!

Did You Know?

If the value of lemons was more known, they would be worth $1.00 each. Lemons are very useful in both health and sickness. Hot lemonade is one of the best remedies for an incipient cold. It is also excellent in cases of biliousness. Lemon syrup, made by baking a lemon 20 minutes then squeezing the juice upon half a cupful of sugar, is excellent for hoarseness and to break up a cold.

Honey is the natural nectar and concentrated sweetness of flowers converted by bees to a golden rich syrup. The sour of nectar the honey is made from determines its color and flavor, and the best is the light-colored variety of honey. The best honey is unadulterated by beekeepers, and is collected from mountainous areas and trees. It is then strained and has most of the impurities removed, except for some pollen and enzymes. Honey is produced by the worker honeybee who sucks flower nectar with its tongue like glossa and stores the nectar in its honey stomach. The bee regurgitates the honey and either stores it in cells or feeds drones. Honey has the ability to absorb and retain moisture, and is an excellent food preservative, and certain varieties of honey are used in treating wounds. (Medicine of the Prophet) Honey should be excluded from the diet of children under the age of one as they are more prone to develop botulism.

Honey contains 35 percent protein (one-half of all the amino acids), and is considered to be a complete food. It is highly concentrated source of essential nutrients, containing large amounts of carbohydrates (sugars), the B-complex vitamins, vitamins C, D, and E, and some minerals. It is used to promote energy and healing. Two tablespoons daily is sufficient. It is twice as sweet as sugar and therefore not as much is needed. Only unfiltered, unheated, unprocessed honey should be purchased. Diabetics and hypoglycemics should be careful when consuming honey and its by-products. The blood sugar reacts to these substances as it would to refined sugars. However, tupelo honey contains more levulose than any other honey and is absorbed at a slower rate so many hypoglycemics can use this type sparingly. (Prescription for Natural Healing, Balch, J. M.D., and Balch,P.A., C.N.C.)

Honey is a natural source of energy that also offers a unique combination of nutritional benefits. Sugars are the fundamental unit of energy for our bodies. All carbohydrates, whether simple sugars or complex carbohydrates, must be broken down to glucose, or blood sugar, before our bodies can use them as energy. The sugars in honey are primarily glucose and fructose and although the body absorbs them in different manners, both provide the body with quick energy. Recent studies suggest that this unique mixture of sugars which occurs naturally in honey, works best in preventing fatigue and enhancing athletic performance. For a quick source of energy and to reap the benefits of honey's healthful properties, make honey part of your daily diet along with plenty of fruits and vegetables. Add honey and fresh fruit to low-fat yogurt for an energy-sustaining snack or stir a spoonful of honey into a glass of water before your daily workout. the ripe fruit of the olive tree of the Oleaceae family. Its native climate is the Mediterranean basin, and its habitat extends throughout the Middle East and Southern Europe, and is found in the North African countries of Morocco and Tunisia as well. (Medicine of the Prophet).

Abu Huraira narrated that Allah's messenger (peace be upon him) said: "Use olive oil as food and as ointment, for it comes from a blessed tree." (Reported by Imam al-Tirmithi.)

Drinking olive oil benefits in the treatment of food poisoning, moves the bowels, and expels intestinal worms. All kinds of oil soften the skin, and slow down the hair graying process. The salted water of preserved olives benefits skin burns, prevents blistering, strengthens the gums, and is good for herpetiform eruptions, and some allergic skin conditions. (Medicine of the Prophet)

Feb 6, 2016 | *Filed under: Featured, Health, Lifestyle, Virtue* | *Posted By MV Media*

By: Healthy Muslim

Black Seeds ... The Islamic Cure

It is narrated by hadith that the Holy Prophet (pbuh) said: "Use the black seed because it has a relief of all diseases, but death." Black seed (Nigella Seed) has a tasty aroma and contains phosphate, iron, phosphorate, carbohydrate, oil 28%. It contains anti-virus bacteria, carotene, anti-cancer fighting material, and hormones which give strength and activity.

FDA Approved Black Seed Oil

In the spring of 1996 the U.S. Food and Drug Administration (FDA) granted a patent for drug use as an immune system stimulant. The drug is based on extracts of "Nigella Sativa," more commonly known as the black seed to Muslims or black cumin. The patent was based on "a pharmaceutical composition containing an extract of the plant Nigella sativa... for treated cancer, preventing the side effects of anticancer chemotherapy, and for increasing the immune functions in humans."

Muslims have been using and promoting the use of the "black seed" or "al-habbatus-sawdaa" for hundreds of years. It has become very popular in recent years and is sold by many Muslim and non-Muslim businesses. A large part of this herbal preparation's popularity is based on the teachings of the Prophet (pbuh).

The Prophet (pbuh) said, "There is healing in the black seed for all diseases except death." However, many products that are presently sold as "black seed" may be black cumin, black caraway, or even coriander. As-Suyuti's Medicine of The Prophet (pbuh) has black seed listed as coriander seeds, with arguments presented for black cumin, terebinth, and even mustard. However, research seems to favor "black cumin" or Nigella sativa as the black seed. Black cumin may be referred to as nutmeg flower or roman coriander, and even fennel flower by gardeners.

Black cumin has been used for a variety of medical problems for several thousand years. They range from stomach aches to asthma, cancer to coughs, and the traditional use as a spice. Black cumin is also used as: a carminative (rids the body of gas from the intestines), a digestive (aids in digestion), a diuretic (increases urine flow by ridding the body of excess water), an emmenagogue (promotes/regulates menstruation), a galactagogue (increases production of milk), a resolvent (dissolves boils & swelling), a stimulant (increases the flow of adrenaline and energy), a stomachic (relieves stomach disorders), a sudorific (increases perspiration), a tonic (improves bodily functions), and a vermifuge (expels worms). Caution should be taken when using the black seed to insure that you are taking the black seed look for the words Nigella sativa. Only this plant, as opposed to true cumin or coriander has the ability to "heal all diseases".

Research suggests that the black seed is an effective anti-tumor treatment for certain types of cancer, including breast cancer and fibrocystic breast disease. The black seed may also be of possible benefit in treating high blood pressure. Except its potential to cause spontaneous abortions (and only in high doses), there may be little, if any, toxic side effects to using it. There is even some research on the possible contraceptive abilities of the black seed. More research is being done on its effectiveness and research trials are also being planned in various countries to study its actual effects on humans. However, the Prophet's (pbuh) words tell us there is healing in this plant. However, there is more to be learned regarding the appropriate doses for various medical problems.

Following are some of the common 'folk remedies' using Black Seed:

1. **Dizziness and ear infection:** use it as a drop for the ears for "infection"; and drink it in tea and rub under your cheek and at the back of your neck for dizziness.

2. **For women and delivery:** it is the best thing for helping with the pains of labor. Boil the black seed with honey and drink.

3. **For skin diseases:** mix a unit of the black seeds' oil with a same unit of rose water and 2 units of brown flour. Before you use the mix rub the area with a cloth dipped in vinegar. Lightly apply the mix to the skin and then expose to the sun every day.

4. **Rheumatism:** Warm black seed oil and massage the oil into the painful areas. Also, make a drink of boiled black seed and mix with honey, drink before going to sleep; and have a lot of yaqeen (full-faith).

5. **High blood pressure:** Mix the black seed with hot liquids you may drink, such as coffee, tea, etc; and rub your body with the oil and have yaqeen.

6. **Chest pains and colds:** Add 1 tablespoon of the black seeds in boiling water and inhale the vapor and cover your head before you sleep.

7. **Heart burn:** add a few drops of black seed oil to a hot cup of milk and add one teaspoon of honey. Also, eat a lot of lettuce.

8. **Eye pain:** rub the oil around the eyes before you sleep and mix a few drops of the oil with hot drinks.

9. **Ulcers:** Mix 10 drops of black seed oil with a cup of honey. Eat 1 spoon of this mixture daily, every morning, before you eat or drink anything else. Follow with a glass of milk. Do this for two months.

10. **Cancer:** Rub the affected area with black seed oil. 3 times a day drink a mixture of a teaspoon of the oil with a glass of carrot juice. Do this for three months.

11. **Laziness:** Mix 10 drops of black seed oil with a glass of orange juice when waking up for 10 days. Important, do not sleep after Fajr salat.

12. **For memorizing:** Boil mint and mix it with honey and 7 drops of black seed oil-drink while warm any time of the day. Also, stop drinking coffee and tea.

Ref: The Islamic Bulletin

10 Natural Remedies for Cold Sores

Cold sores are painful blisters around the corners of your lips, caused by the herpes simplex virus (HSV). There are two different types of herpes simplex viruses, which are known as the HSV-1 and HSV-2 strains. The virus usually enters the body through a break in the skin and is extremely contagious. The most common symptoms include a burning or tingling sensation in or outside of the mouth, which eventually turns into a blister that goes away within a few days. The blister goes from a bright red color to a crusty yellow scab before falling off. You can speed up the healing process with a few natural home remedies listed below:

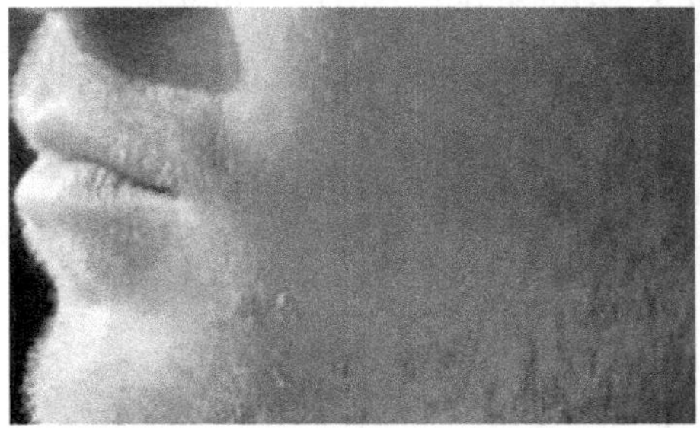

The Most Common Causes & Symptoms: Causes:

- Hormonal changes (especially during menstruation)
- Emotional stress
- Fever
- Trauma to the skin (such as a fall)
- Long exposure to sunlight

Symptoms:

- Pain around your mouth and on your lips
- Fever
- Sore throat
- Swollen glands in your neck or other parts of the body.

10 Natural Remedies to Treat Cold Sores:

1. **Cold Milk -** A glass of cold milk can help sooth the tingling sensation and discomfort caused by the virus. Whole milk contains immunoglobulins, which prevent the cold sores from spreading.

   Remedy:

   - Soak a cotton ball in cold, whole milk.
   - Apply it on the cold sore and leave it on for around 10 minutes.
   - Repeat the process twice daily.

2. **Lemon Balm -** Lemon balm prevents the cold sores from spreading, since it contains polyphenolic compounds and tannins that add to its antiviral effects.

   Remedy:

   - Steep one to two teaspoons of dried lemon balm leaves in one liter (or 4 cups) of hot water for 10 minutes.
   - Strain and drink three to four cups of this herbal tea with each meal throughout the day.

- Apply lemon balm tea or essential oil on your cold sore three to five times a day, and repeat until blisters go away.

3. **Ice -** Ice provides a temporary relief from the painful sores by reducing the redness and swelling. Ice cools off the blister and prevents it from growing to a larger size.

   Remedy:

   - Take a single ice cube and wrap it inside a clean washcloth.
   - Place the washcloth over your cold sore for about 10 to 15 minutes.
   - Repeat the process every three to four hours or until blister reduces.

4. **Echinacea -** The powerful herb contains many antiviral properties, while keeping your immune system fully protected. Echinacea extract is also used to treat herpes simplex virus-1.

   Remedy:

   - Dab Echinacea liquid extract on the affected area.
   - You can drink Echinacea tea, in the form of tincture or capsules. Consult your doctor before taking any capsules or if you're currently on any particular medications.
   - Do not take the herb for more than eight weeks.

5. **Licorice Root -** Licorice contains the glycyrrhizic acid ingredient, which is used to treat the sores. Chew on a few sticks of the snack treat for temporary pain relief or use the root powder as a topical solution.

   Remedy:

   - Mix one tablespoon of licorice root powder and one-half teaspoon of water.
   - Apply the mixture on the cold sore using a cotton swab or your fingertip.
   - Allow it to stay for a few hours.
   - Repeat several times throughout the day.
   - Alternatively, You can chew on natural licorice sticks, drink licorice root tea or take them in supplement form. Make sure you consult your physician before taking any supplements.

6. **Hydrogen Peroxide -** Hydrogen peroxide can be applied after the sore has turned into a yellowish blister, as a cleansing antiseptic. Do not use the peroxide on a red blister, since it can severely aggravate it. Use the peroxide during the blister phase or the early scab phase.

   Remedy:

   - Dip a cotton swab in 3% hydrogen peroxide solution.
   - Apply it on the cold sore area, and leave it on for a few minutes.
   - Repeat every couple of hours.

7. **Tea Tree Oil -** The antiviral properties found in tea tree oil can reduce the cold sore by nearly half its original size overnight. The oil also contains antiseptic, anti-fungal and anti-inflammatory components, all essential for treating the red blisters.

   Remedy:

   - Add three parts of water to one part of tea tree oil in order to dilute it.
   - Dip a cotton ball in the tea tree oil and apply it on the affected area three times a day.

- You can also combine tea tree oil with an equal amount of olive oil and a little eucalyptus oil, and apply as a topical treatment two to three times a day.

8. **Acetone Nail Polish Remover -** Who would ever guess that a little dab of nail polish remover would make such a useful cold sore remedy? The acetone works to get rid of the discomfort and dry the cold sore faster.

Remedy:

- Dip a cotton ball into the nail polish remover.
- Dab the cotton ball on the affected area.
- Repeat several times a day, preferably once an hour.

9. **Garlic -** The powerful enzymes contained in garlic, act as antibacterial, antifungal and antiviral agents, which help treat the blisters. Garlic reduces swelling and inflammation, while increasing the healing process.

Remedy:

- Cut a clove of garlic into halves.
- Crush one-half of the garlic and apply it on the affected area.
- Allow the garlic to stand for 10 to 15 minutes.
- Repeat the process about three to five times a day.

10. **Lysine -** Lysine blocks the activity of an amino acid called arginine, which triggers the herpes simplex virus. You can either consume the essential amino acid through products, such as milk, soybeans, and cheese or in supplement form.

Remedy:

- Include a diet of protein-rich foods, such as; cheese, milk, meat, yogurt, and soybeans.
- You can Take 1,000 to 1,500 mg L-Lysine supplements daily to help treat the herpes virus and 1,000 mg three times a day or during an outbreak. Consult with your doctor before taking any supplements.

Bonus Tips:

- Avoid acidic foods, such as; citrus fruits, tomatoes and anything with vinegar.
- Avoid stress.
- Avoid picking at it to minimize the risks for infection.
- Limit your exposure to the sun, since it can cause cold sores to flare.
- Use lip balm and sunscreen on your face when it gets hot outside.
- Wash your hands thoroughly.
- Avoid sharing towels, razors, silverware, and toothbrushes, which other people with the illness might have used.
- Avoid contact with people that have been infected with the disease.
- Don't share eating utensils that an infected person might have used before.

H/T: top10homeremedies.com

9 Natural Remedies For Nausea

Nausea is that unpleasant feeling of discomfort inside your stomach, oftentimes leading to vomiting. The most common causes for nausea can stem from food poisoning, side effects of certain medications, pregnancy, ulcers, motion sickness, and acid reflux digestion problems.

You don't need to head out to the doctor's office when you hear a rumbling in your stomach. There are plenty of natural remedies that can be found at home that can treat nausea. Here are 10 natural cures for nausea that will help soothe your stomach:

1. **Ginger** - Ginger is a powerful ingredient that's helpful in many situations. Adding ginger to a cup of hot tea can work wonders for an upset stomach. You can also drink Ginger Ale if you have any in your fridge, or make it from scratch (recipe listed below). Ginger promotes the secretion of various digestive juices and enzymes, which neutralizes stomach acid.

   ### Directions For Making Ginger Tea:

   - 1 ginger root
   - 2-3 cups of water
   - Honey (optional but recommended)
   - Wax paper
   - A cutting board

   How To Prepare It:
   Make sure you thoroughly wash the ginger to get all the bacteria out. You will then want to slice the ginger into tiny pieces. Place a cover with wax paper over the sliced ginger and crush it. Boil 2-3 cups of water over a medium-high flame before adding the ginger. Allow the ginger to boil between 3-5 minutes. Remove the concoction from the heat and pour everything into a tea cup. You can also strain it before pouring it into the cup. Honey can increase the flavor, and help keep the nausea at bay. Find a comfortable chair, sit down, sip slowly and relax.

   ### Directions For Making Ginger Ale:

   - Add 2 cups of chopped ginger roots
   - Add 3-4 strips of lemon or lime peels
   - Add 3 quarts of chilled club soda
   - Add 1/2 cup of sugar
   - Add several ice cubes

   How To Prepare It:
   Add 2 cups of freshly peeled and chopped gingerroot with lemon or lime peel, and 4 cups of water. Let the mix boil over a high flame, and then at an active simmer. Let the Ginger Ale remain uncovered for 10 minutes. Add some sugar while stirring, and continue to boil the mixture for about 15 minutes or so. Strain the ginger syrup over a large bowl, separating the ginger roots from the liquid mixture. Use a glass container to chill the syrup until cold, or up to a week. Mix 1/4 cup of the syrup with 1 cup of the cold club soda and pour over ice.

2. **Eat Some Milk Toast** - Toast is an ideal food to digest for treating stomach disorders. Bread helps absorb excess stomach acid, which can trigger nausea and vomiting. The milk helps coat your stomach. Milk toast is very easy to make and very effective once consumed. DO NOT consume if you have gastroenteritis.

   ### Directions For Making Milk Toast:

   - 1 cup of milk
   - 1 piece of toast
   - Some unsalted butter

How To Prepare It:

Heat a cup of milk up, but make sure the milk is not boiling. Pour the milk into a small cereal bowl, and let it cool off for a few moments. Put the bread into the toaster, and spread a tiny bit of unsalted butter on it. Crush the toast into the milk, and eat slowly. Drink the tea with ginger after you've eaten the toast to soothe the stomach acids.

3. **Smell a Sliced Lemon or Peppermint Oil** - You would never think that the scents of peppermint oil and lemons could help cure nausea, but they do. The strong citrus scents in the lemon helps to soothe your stomach, while the peppermint oil can be gently rubbed onto your gums with your fingertips.
The lemon should be sliced in half before inhaling the citrus aromas. Lemon juice can also be extracted into your ginger tea for a great taste. You can keep a few wedges of lemon or lime in a Ziploc Bag in the freezer, and suck on the frozen cirtrus fruits to reduce nausea.

4. **Use A Cold Compress On Your Neck** - Grab an ice pack from the freezer, but make sure it stays out for a few minutes before applying it on your neck. Apply the cool compress to the back of your neck to help reduce the nausea levels. If you don't have any ice pack, you can simply take a cold washcloth dipped in cool water and follow the same protocol.

5. **Stay On A BRAT Diet** - B.R.A.T is an acronym for Bananas, Rice, Applesauce and Toast. These bland foods are low in fiber to limit any gastrointestinal disorders. If you're well enough to eat, you can start by consuming any of the above mentioned foods/ Remember to eat very slowly.

6. **Avoid Dehydration** - You lose a large volume of fluid and electrolytes during a stomach virus or after you vomit. It's essential to replace the lost fluids to prevent dehydration from occurring. Make sure you drink plenty of cold water, but drink it in tiny sips. Alternatively, you can sip on some sports drinks to regain the lost electrolytes and stay fully hydrated.

7. **Get Some Air** - It's crucial to step outside and breathe some fresh air. You can also open the windows to air out the house or sit on the balcony if you're too ill to walk far. If you're feeling a bit flushed, you can turn the fan on. Just make sure you keep it on a low speed.

8. **Go To Bed** - Go to the bedroom, and pull the shades down so that it's dark and cool in the room. Lie down with your head on a single flat pillow and keep your knees bent to prevent any pressure to your stomach area. Regularly breathe to avoid any stress, which could worsen the nausea.

9. **Stretch** - A discomforting feeling in the upper back or neck region can trigger vomiting and nausea. Try doing some simple neck and back stretches in orde to alleviate the tension that is causing the upset stomach.

A Stretching Exerise For The Back:

Place a yoga mat or a towel down on the floor, and position your body as if you're about to do a push-up. Lift your upper body up, and arch your back as you tilt the head back as far as possible, the underneath of your chin facing the ceiling. Your body should form a "U" position.

A Stretching Exercise For The Neck:

Sit on a chair and tip your head forward, while touching your chin to your chest. Hold the stretch for about 10-15 seconds. It's important that you tilt NOT roll the neck to prevent pinched nerves or induce the nausea. Tilt your head to left, as if you're trying to touch your ear to your shoulder. Hold the stretch for 10-15 seconds, before repeating to the other side.

Ref: http://www.ba-bamail.com/

8 Natural Ways to Get Rid of Gingivitis

Gingivitis is a gum disease that is more common than you think. Anyone can get it. Bacteria that sit in your mouth can lead to plaque formation, which is a sticky film that irritates the gums and teeth. It's a mild disease and is characterized by redness, swelling, irritation and puffy gums. In the early stages most people don't know that they even have it. It can lead to gum recession along with loose teeth and bad breath. Here are some natural home remedies that can help you get rid of this annoying disease.

1. Tea tree oil

Tea tree oil is well known for oral health benefits and is a natural antibiotic and anti-inflammatory. Studies have found those with chronic gingivitis who brushed their teeth using tea tree oil toothpaste, had their inflammation reduced by half. It's important not to apply tea tree oil directly to the gums or swallow it in its pure form. it can irritate the gums and can cause diarrhea.
The best way to use this essential oil for your gums is by buying a special tea tree oil toothpaste, or adding a drop of tea tree oil to your regular toothpaste every time you brush your teeth.

2. Peppermint

A natural way to treat your gums for gingivitis is with peppermint due to it being antibacterial and antiseptic. Applying peppermint to your teeth and gums also reduces any inflammation and removes bacteria that cause bad breath. You can crush peppermint leaves and soak them in water for thirty minutes. Use this solution as a mouthwash and rinse your mouth with it three times daily. Another way to apply peppermint is by drinking a strong cup of peppermint tea between meals. Alternatively brush your teeth and gums with a peppermint-flavored toothpaste.

3. Salt

This mineral with its antiseptic and antibacterial properties is effective in treating gum disease. The salt can treat any swollen or inflamed gums, draw infections out of abscesses and stop the growth of bacteria. The best way to apply salt is by rinsing your mouth with a saline salt mix twice daily. Add half a teaspoon of salt to a glass of lukewarm water and rinse in the mornings and evenings. Another way to apply it is by making a paste with mustard oil. Add half a teaspoon of salt to mustard oil. Use as much oil needed until a paste forms. Massage this treatment into the gums using circular strokes for two minutes. Then gargle with warm water. Repeat this treatment twice daily until you notice results, which should be within a few days.

4. Guava leaves

Dental studies have found that those with low vitamin C levels experience more gum disease. Traditionally 18th century sailors used to eat limes, a fruit high in vitamin C, to prevent bleeding gums. Although limes and oranges are high in vitamin C, an antioxidant which accelerates bone regeneration and helps repair connective tissues, guavas have higher amounts of the vitamin. Guava leaves are also anti-inflammatory, antimicrobial and have analgesic properties. Guaijaverin, a plant flavonoid found in the leaves, is an effective antiplaque agent.
You can rinse your mouth with the leaves by chewing them and spitting them out. If this sounds unpleasant, you can grind the leaves and add it to your toothpaste, or buy mouthwash with guava leaf extract.

5. Lemon juice

Although guavas have higher dosages of vitamin C, lemon juice is easier to locate all year round. Lemons also contain antibacterial and anti-inflammatory properties that can help with gum disease. You can mix lemon juice with a glass of warm water and use this as a mouthwash. Rinse your mouth with this solution after brushing your teeth. Alternatively you can make a paste with one tablespoon lemon juice and salt, and apply it to your gums, leaving it on for five minutes. Rinse off the paste with warm water and repeat four times a day until you notice an improvement.

6. Turmeric

Turmeric contains lots of curcumin, a natural anti-inflammatory, and antioxidant. This effectively lessens plaque, pain, swelling and gum inflammation. Curcumin also reduces bacterial activity, which prevents infection. Periodontists have found turmeric to be as effective as a traditional chlorhexidine mouthwash in fighting plaque, inflammation, and bacteria. You can apply turmeric as a paste: Mix one teaspoon turmeric powder with half a teaspoon of salt, and half a teaspoon of mustard oil. Apply and massage on your teeth and gums twice a day.
Another way to apply it is by making a gum pack. Mix half a teaspoon turmeric powder to a little water or vitamin E oil and apply this on your gums for ten minutes. Rinse with warm water, once a day for several weeks. Alternatively you can make a paste of turmeric powder and a bit of water and brush it on your teeth with a soft- bristle toothbrush. This can be done twice a day for a few weeks.

Ref: http://www.ba-bamail.com/

12 Home Remedies for a Toothache

There is nothing quite as painful and frustrating as a toothache. The good news is that you can treat the toothache with a dozen natural home remedies to help alleviate the pain. There's also a very good chance that you have most of the items on the list inside your fridge, or kitchen cabinet drawers.

A toothache is the result of an irritated or inflamed pulp, which is situated within the central region of the tooth. The sensitive nerve endings inside the pulp can get triggered by foods or beverages that are either too cold or too hot. It's important to first get a better understanding of the most common causes and symptoms before you begin the home remedies.

NOTE: None of these are a replacement for an actual dentist. These remedies will help you pass the time until your dentist appointment or alleviate some of the pain after, but do not skip the dentist visit. Teeth problems are serious health problems and should be treated as such.

Causes of Tooth Pain:

- Abscessed tooth
- Infected gums (gingivitis)
- Tooth decay
- Damaged fillings
- Dental injuries, such as a chipped or fractured tooth
- Sinus infection
- Wisdom teeth
- Temporomandibular Joint Syndrome (TMJ)

Symptoms of Tooth Pain:

- Swelling around the tooth
- Fever
- Headache
- Foul-tasting drainage from the infected tooth
- Sharp pain when pressure is applied to tooth
- Sensitivity to hot or cold foods

12 Natural Home Remedies for a Toothache:

1. **Cloves -** When it comes to natural home remedies for tooth infections, there is nothing that ranks higher than cloves! Cloves contain extremely powerful antibacterial, anti-inflammatory, and anesthetic properties that help alleviate tooth pain. The anesthetic properties also help to fight off the infection.

   ### The Remedy:

   - Take a pair of cloves and grind them with a little mix of olive oil or vegetable oil.
   - Apply the clove solution onto the affected tooth.
   - Dab clove oil solution onto a cotton ball, and rub directly on the affected tooth.
   - You can also mix a few drops of clove oil in half a glass of water, and use it as a mouthwash after the dabbing process.

2. **Warm Salt Water -** All it takes is a glass of warm water mixed with a bit of salt, and you can reduce the pain of a toothache. This homemade mouthwash solution will assist in fighting bacteria that causes tooth decay and infection.

   ### The Remedy:

   - Mix half a spoon of common salt in a glass of very warm water.

- Gargle thoroughly with the warm salt water solution.
- Repeat a few times, or until you feel better.

3. **Ice Cube** - Head over to the freezer and pull out a couple of ice cubes. The ice cube helps numb the infected nerves that cause the horrible pain. Dentists use ice to test for sensitivity on teeth as well.

The Remedy:

- Place an ice cube inside a Ziploc bag and wrap it in a thin cotton cloth.
- Hold the bag over your cheek near the aching tooth for a couple of minutes.
- The ice will then indicate the exposed nerves. Take a bit of caution when applying the ice.

4. **Salt and Pepper** - The next remedy can be found on your kitchen table. Salt and pepper provide a wonderful relief when combined together. The natural antibiotics inside the mouthwash can help ease the uncomfortable pain within the pulp region.

The Remedy:

- Mix equal amounts of regular table salt and pepper with a few drops of water. This will form a natural kind of paste.
- Apply the paste directly on the tooth, and allow the paste to take effect for a couple of minutes.
- Repeat process for a few days, or until tooth feels better.

5. **Garlic** - It's no secret that garlic is the "cure-all" when it comes to home remedies. Garlic is not only ideal for treating a common old, but also for treating toothaches. Garlic contains a bunch of antibiotic properties that can help get rid of tooth pain.

The Remedy:

- Mix a clove of crushed garlic or use some garlic powder together with a sprinkle of table salt, and apply to the painful tooth.
- You can even chew on a few cloves of garlic for some quick relief.
- Continue the garlic remedy for several days, or until pain stops.

6. **Asafetida** - The powdered gum resin inside the Asafetida can help reduce pain during a toothache, and for bleeding gums. The odor of the Asafetida might not be too pleasant, but the natural pain remedy is worth the bad smell!

The Remedy:

- Add a pinch of powdered Asafetida with lemon juice.
- Warm up the solution, and use a cotton pad to apply the mixture on the affected area.
- Asafetida can also be fried in clarified butter, and placed inside the tooth cavity for instant relief.

7. **Baking Soda** - Baking soda helps whiten your teeth and acts as a natural painkiller for toothaches, when mixed together with a bit of water. Baking soda promotes quicker healing of painful or swollen gum tissues, which is the reason why many toothpastes feature the sodium bicarbonate on the labels.

The Remedy:

- Take a cotton swab and moisten it with a bit of water.
- Dip the wet cotton swab in baking soda. Coat the swab really well so that it absorbs the baking soda before applying to infected tooth.
- A mouth rinse can be made by mixing a large spoonful of baking soda into a small glass of warm water. Let the baking soda dissolve before swishing the rinse in your mouth.

8. **Lime or Lime Juice -** The citric acid of the lime juice helps kill the germs that cause tooth infection. Lime juice also contains vitamin C, which keeps your teeth protected against decay. Mixing lime juice and baking soda can also help whiten teeth.

The Remedy: Lime Juice

- Combine the lime juice together with Asafetida to form a paste.
- Apply the lime paste on the infected tooth.
- Keep your mouth slightly open to allow the paste to dry on the tooth.
- Apply the paste 2-3 times a day to reduce the pain.

Limes

- Cut a lime wedge or slice, and bite directly into it. Try to extract some of the juice.
- Allow the lime to sit outside for a bit if you're feeling any sensitivity to cold.
- Repeat process as needed, or until pain goes away.

9. **Vanilla Extract -** Vanilla extract contains Eugenol, which has antiseptic and analgesic properties that are used to fight off tooth decay. The Eugenol helps get rid of that unwanted toothache, and provides a quick pain relief solution.

The Remedy:

- Saturate a cotton swab or cotton ball with 3-4 drops of vanilla extract, and place on affected tooth.
- Use your finger to rub the vanilla extract on the affected area. Make sure you wash your hands thoroughly beforehand.
- Repeat process until pain goes away.

10. **Onion -** Onions offer great pain relief to people suffering from tooth abscesses or sensitive gums. Onions are highly regarded by dentists for their natural and powerful antimicrobial properties. Onions have even been compared to taking 8 Advil capsules, or an entire bottle of Orajel!

The Remedy:

- Slice a piece of fresh onion and hold it inside your mouth.
- Gently bite the onion until the juices come out for a few minutes to alleviate pain.
- You may also put a piece of onion on the painful tooth so that it absorbs the antiseptic and antimicrobial properties.
- Continue process until pain reduces.

11. **Bayberry -** The root bark of the bayberry is used to help strengthen gums. The berries are ideal for treating aching wisdom teeth as well. The natural antibiotics of the bayberry should go to work very quickly on your aching tooth.

The Remedy:

- Mix the bayberry bark together with vinegar to form a natural paste.
- Apply the paste on the affected tooth as a pain relief.
- Use the paste when needed, or several times per day.

12. **Guava Leaves -** Guava leaves are used to heal mouth sores and aching teeth. The juice of the guava leaves contains many antibacterial properties that thwart off tooth decay or gingivitis. You should feel the effects of the guava leaves shortly after applying to the sensitive areas.

The Remedy:

- Chew on a couple of guava leaves until the juice begins to work on the affected tooth.
- Place 4 to 5 guava leaves in water and let it boil.
- Allow the solution to cool off a bit before adding a pinch of salt, and rinse your mouth thoroughly with

it. Ref: (H/T: top10homeremedies.com)

The Best Home Remedies for Chest Congestion

Chest congestion is an unpleasant inflammation of the lower respiratory system that can make your breathing become difficult and painful. In many cases, it is caused by common conditions, such as colds and respiratory infections. In order to prevent any complications, it is important to clear it before it worsens. Here are some natural home remedies for chest congestion that can help you alleviate the symptoms and return you to your previous, congestion-free, health.

What is Chest Congestion

Chest congestion is the accumulation of excess fluid and mucus (a slippery secretion produced by the respiratory membranes – also referred to as snot or phlegm) in the lungs. It is a symptom of many illnesses, some benign and some of a more serious type. For the latter, a visit to the doctor is always recommended, so that you receive the right treatment timely.

The most common symptoms of chest congestion include:

- cough
- difficulty breathing and shortness of breath
- pain in the chest
- dizziness
- runny nose

If you don't have any concerns regarding the origin of your congestion and it can be attributed to the common cold or the flu, it's best to try and treat it naturally before reaching for the artificial chemical substances.

How to Get Rid of Chest Congestion Naturally

Increase your fluid intake

Drinking plenty of fluids is essential. It helps the body stay hydrated (when you're ill, you're more likely to suffer dehydration) and thins the mucus, so it's easier to cough it out. In addition to pure water, drink herbal teas. Chamomile and ginger teas can be particularly soothing. According to <u>WebMD</u> (and many mothers and grandmothers), consuming hot chicken soup also does the trick. Some studies suggest that the soup helps activate the disease-fighting white blood cells and improves the function of protective structures inside the lungs.

<u>Fluids to avoid:</u>

- Alcoholic beverages
- Caffeinated drinks (coffee, black tea, sodas)
- Drinks with high sugar content

Use Steam and Essential Oils
Steam, too, will help you soften the mucus and clear your chest. It can be used in different ways:

- Steam vaporizer – If you have access to one, use it to create warm and humid conditions in your room during the night.
- Hot showers – Treat yourself to a steamy shower or sit in the bathroom whilst a hot shower is running.
- Steam inhalations – This is my favorite steaming method. Boil some water and pour it into a bowl. Add a few drops of essential oils (good for congestion are eucalyptus, <u>peppermint</u>, rosemary, <u>tea tree</u> and thyme oils). Then, cover your head with a large towel, lean over the bowl and inhale for 10 minutes or more.
- Sauna – If you can, and your condition is not contagious, visit to a steam sauna might be beneficial and will help ease the congestion, as well as detox the whole body.

Spice up your meals

- Garlic – Garlic is one of my favorite home remedies and it's also one of the herbs I mentioned in my e-Book **The**

<u>**Herbal Remedies Guide**</u>. Add garlic to your food or eat it raw. This natural antibiotic acts in an anti-microbial way and boosts the immune system. Pay special attention to avoid these <u>6 common mistakes when using garlic as a medicine</u>. Garlic is also one of the ingredients in my homemade <u>natural syrup for chest infections</u>.

- <u>Ginger</u> – You can eat it raw, make a hot drink or use it as a spice. You can also combine it with some other spices to make a delicious and potent beverage. Try adding a teaspoon of ginger to a cup of hot water and add some ground cloves and cinnamon. Sweeten with raw honey.

- Chili peppers – Full of antioxidants, they will provide a kick to your meal and act as a natural decongestant and expectorants (aiding the clearance of mucus).

- Turmeric – This anti-inflammatory 'king of spices' should also be included in your diet. Make a hot drink such as this <u>turmeric golden milk</u> or prepare a more exotic meal. Turmeric has low absorption and rapid metabolism but there are <u>natural ways to improve its absorption in your body</u>.

Drink hot tea with lemon and honey

This is one of the simplest home remedies that will help you relieve the symptoms and up your fluid intake. The vitamin C in lemons helps strengthen the immune system, while honey has anti-viral and anti-microbial properties. You can also <u>use honey and lemon in many other ways to improve your health</u>.

Use apple cider vinegar

You might not like the taste, but <u>ACV</u> will improve your breathing and deal with bacteria that cause the extra mucus. You can combine it with some turmeric and add <u>raw honey</u> to improve the taste. Drink a shot every 8 hours, but don't overdo it or you might end up with an upset stomach.

You can also try this combination of ACV and honey (which is also helpful for <u>sinus infections</u>):

- a glass of warm water

- 1 teaspoon of honey

- 1 tablespoon of apple cider vinegar

Make a hot pack

Put a steaming hot cloth on your chest and throat and leave it there for 10 to 15 minutes (lay down with your head elevated). You can also roast some fenugreek, cloves and carom (ajwain) seeds and put them in a cloth to create a pack that will provide you with immense relief.

Some More Natural Expectorants

1. Horseradish – WebMD also recommends using horseradish, which contains a chemical similar to pharmaceutical decongestants. You can find more information on how to use horseradish as a medicine in <u>this article</u>.

2. Fennel – This spice will naturally move mucus from your lungs. You can use sautéed fennel or mix it with some curry powder.

3. Gargle salt water – To get rid of mucus, gargle for 1 to 2 minutes a mixture of warm water and salt. You can also add turmeric to saline water.

How To Prevent Chest Congestion

To stay clear of chest infections, do the following:

- Exercise – this will help with the health of your lungs, breathing muscles and air circulation.
- Get enough sleep.
- Practice a relaxation technique (<u>yoga</u>, <u>meditation</u>, mindfulness).
- Stay sufficiently hydrated.

- Limit unhealthy fats, salt and processed foods – enjoy a balanced diet.

- Avoid foods that produce mucus: dairy products, salt, sugar, fried foods.

- Get enough vitamin D and sun exposure. A <u>lack of vitamin D can cause 12 common diseases</u>.

- Stop smoking. You can get advice on how to quit smoking in my article about the <u>5 natural ways to quit smoking</u>.

- Avoid taking suppressants – These are drugs that stop you coughing. But, at the same time, they thicken mucus in your chest and keep it there where it can become a breeding ground for infections. When you have chest congestion, you need to cough to get the lungs clear again, so don't try to stop the body's natural mechanisms.

Ref: Healthy and Natural World

Home Remedies for Hair Loss

Hair loss is normal, but when it happens in excess it's frightening and upsetting. It's common to lose about 50-100 strands a day, and up to 250 strands when you wash your hair. About 10% of your hair is dormant, and will fall out after 2-3 months. Sometimes you may not realize that everyday habits can contribute to hair loss. Here are some natural ways to promote hair growth and prevent hair loss, as well as some tips on what not to do to ensure that your hair stays on your head.

Home Remedies:

1. **Coconut milk**

   Coconut milk contains a rich source of nutrients including vitamin E, potassium, and iron. Applying this liquid directly to the roots can help prevent hair breakage and accelerate hair growth. The antibacterial properties in the milk can also protect the scalp as it is a natural conditioner for both hair and skin. It's recommended that you leave the treatment in overnight.

2. **Amla, Indian gooseberry**

   This fruit is well known for its high levels of vitamins. It is also packed with antioxidants, which can prevent premature graying of the hair. The essential fatty acids in this fruit can also keep hair follicles strong. Apply a paste of dried amla with lime juice to the scalp to nourish your locks and make your hair extra lustrous. To make the paste mix 2 teaspoons of lime juice with 2 teaspoons of dried amla powder.

3. **Scalp massage**

   Regularly treating your head to a massage is effective in keeping your hair healthy. A massage stimulates blood flow to the scalp and promotes hair growth. Combining a head massage with lukewarm oil can prevent hair loss and dandruff too.
   There are a number of oils to try: coconut, jojoba, mustard, almond, lavender, olive, or sesame oil - all full of added nutrients. Jojoba oil is especially recommended because it replaces sebum (an oily secretion from the sevaceous glands) in the scalp.

4. **Neem, Indian lilac**

   Neem oil is extracted from the fruit of the Indian lilac tree. This treatment is effective because the tree is rich in antioxidants which counter free radicals. Neem is regenerative and contains fatty acids like linoleic, oleic, and stearic acids, which also condition the scalp and hair.
   Neem is an astringent and can also treat itching, dandruff and head lice without chemicals. Neem oil has a bitter smell so it's recommended that you mix it with an aromatic essential oil like lavender, tea tree or orange. You can massage this mixture into your scalp and apply it to your locks too.

5. **Aloe vera**

   Aloe Vera is another good remedy for hair loss. Applying pure aloe gel directly to the scalp helps balance the pH level. The plant extract is rich in vitamins, amino acids, minerals, and enzymes. The aloe strengthens hair elasticity and can soften and moisturize your hair, acting as a natural conditioner. Dissolving a small amount of salt into the gel can also help. The salt penetrates through deeper skin layers and can prevent hair from falling out unnecessarily.

6. **Egg white and curd**

   The combination of egg white and curd creates a super hair treatment that promotes hair growth. Eggs are rich in sulfur, selenium, iodine, phosphorus, iron and zinc. Curd has many nutrients and is anti-fungal. This mixture makes an excellent conditioner, making your hair look shiny and at the same time, it effectively fights dandruff and hair loss. Combine the ingredients and apply the mask to your scalp and hair.

7. Henna

While most people know henna as a natural hair dye, it is also an excellent way to strengthen and condition your hair. More importantly henna controls excessive hair loss. When applied to the hair and scalp it creates a protective coat over the hair shafts and its nutrients repair the hair cuticles, making the strands thick and strong. To prevent hair loss, combine dried henna leaves or powdered henna with mustard oil and a teaspoon of lemon juice. Massage this oil mix into your scalp. Leave it to rest for 30 minutes and rinse your hair after.

8. Hibiscus

This vibrant flower has many rejuvenating properties for hair. It is an old Indian method of maintaining a thick mane of hair. Because of its rich vitamin C and amino acid content, this flower works to prevent premature graying. It also nourishes the hair and treats dandruff. When you combine the crushed leaves of the flowers with coconut or sesame oil and apply this paste to your scalp regularly, it can help with hair loss. It's best to leave the paste in your hair for several hours and then rinse.

Habits to avoid:

Don't comb or rub your hair while wet
Wet hair is more fragile because the protective layer has been stripped. Towel drying or combing your hair when wet can cause the hair to snap and break. Untangle your hair before you wet it and blot your hair with a towel.

Don't overheat your hair
Excess use of your hair dryer or straightening iron can dry out your hair shafts, leading to dull, and brittle hair. The heat can damage the proteins and the dryness also strips your hair of natural moisture, resulting in dry cuticles, which will snap off. It's recommended you limit this activity to 2 to 3 times a week.

Don't wash your hair with hot water
Boiling hot water can weaken your hair follicles and cause hair to fall out. Having a steaming hot shower frequently can strip away the protective oils and this can cause your scalp pores to overproduce oil, which can damage the hair at the root, resulting in excessive shedding. Opt for washing your hair with lukewarm to warm water, and rinsing with cooler temperatures, to lock in moisture.

H/T: www.stylecraze.com

Home Remedies To Control Blood Sugar Levels

Diabetes is one of the leading concerns among health professionals today, as more and more individuals fall prey to this life-long and dangerous disease. It is caused when the blood sugar levels rise to an excess, which results in a resistance to insulin. Once this happens, the diabetic individual can no longer control their blood sugar levels, and they can rise and fall with serious consequences. Yet whether you are diabetic or know someone diabetic or not, it is important to implement measures to control blood sugar levels and to stop the spread of diabetes in its tracks.

1. **Consume More Dairy Products**

    The protein and fat in dairy products helps improve blood sugar levels, and if the products are low in fat, it has been shown that they can also decrease the chances for developing insulin resistance.

2. **Choose the Right Kind of Bread**

    Avoid white flour based products at all costs! These simple carbohydrates are full of sugar that spike up your blood sugar. Instead, you should consume whole wheat or rye products that are high in fiber, protein and complex carbohydrates, which control blood glucose levels and keep you full longer.

3. **Maximize the Magnesium**

    Magnesium is a mineral known to help prevent the onset of Type II diabetes and should be consumed as much as possible. It is best to consume natural sources of magnesium such as spinach, fish, nuts, leafy greens and avocados. All of these foods have been proven to lower the risk of diabetes and can even aid in weight loss.

4. **Cardamom is great!**

    Cardamom is a member of the ginger family of spices and comes from Asia as well as South America. The spice is known to regulate Type II diabetes and can be sprinkled on coffee, tea, yogurt and even cereal. The spice is known to help decrease blood glucose levels by eighteen to thirty percent.

5. **Buckwheat**

    Buckwheat is an excellent source of fiber that you may have never heard of. It also does wonders for maintaining healthy blood sugar levels. Buckwheat comes in the form of soba noodles, which are a delicious substitute for rice or pasta, as well as in a number of powders that can be added to baked goods or even on top of a slice of (whole wheat) bread.

6. **Drink in Moderation**

    Alcohol contains huge amounts of sugar, and anyone trying to watch out for their blood sugar should definitely moderate the amount of alcohol they consume. It is best to occasionally drink wine with dinner, and not after dinner when the same glass of wine could alter insulin levels in the blood.

7. **Watch Fat Intake**

    It is important to watch the amount of saturated fats entering the body because these can seriously increase the chances of contracting diabetes. Saturated fats are usually found in fried and junk foods as they are cooked in unhealthy oils.

8. **Exercise Daily**

    Getting in exercise each day is critical to maintaining normal blood sugar levels, even if it's a brisk walk in the park.

9. Laughing

Yes, this really is one of the tips that will lower your chances of developing diabetes. It was found that those who laugh have lower blood sugar levels than those who don't laugh enough
(this means you should keep reading our jokes!).

10. Eat Grapefruit

Grapefruit has been proven to aid in weight loss as it affects the glucose metabolism, keeping insulin levels steady.

11. Do Resistance Training

Building muscle mass is important for burning more glucose out of your system. Training once to twice a week could significantly aid in preventing the occurrence of diabetes.

12. Drink Decaf, Not Regular

Decaffeinated coffee slows down the rate at which the intestines absorb sugars and speeds up the absorption of sugar by the muscles.

13. Eat Smaller Meals

It is best to have a small meal and then another small meal (or a second half of the regular sized meal) later on (at half hour intervals). It is also important to eat regularly so that insulin levels don't spike, but remain stable throughout the day.

14. Get Enough Sleep

Sleep deprivation can affect blood sugar and insulin levels so it is important to get enough sleep each night. It is also essential to stop snoring because according to some studies, those who snore are more likely to develop diabetes (because snoring is often tied to being overweight).

15. Learn Relaxation

Listen to soothing music or read an interesting book, whatever you need to do to relax. Meditation and yoga can also help if they are done properly and on a regular basis.

Ref: http://www.ba-bamail.com/

10 Remedies for Dark Circles and Puffy Eyes

One of the main reasons that we get dark circles around are eyes is genetics, but also getting older, dry skin, crying, long hours facing a computer screen, stress, lack of sleep and an unhealthy diet. Men and women from different age groups can suffer from this problem, and even though it's not a health risk, no one looks to look exhausted and tired.Luckily, there are a number of handy home remedies that'll get rid of those dark shadows with a few common ingredients found in any home.

1. Turmeric

Turmeric has both antioxidants and anti-inflammation properties and so can be used to freshen your skin and fix that tired look. Take the powder and mix it with pineapple water to create a thick mix. Smear the mix under your eyes, leave for 10 minutes and then wipe with a moist, soft cloth. Aside from removing the circles, it will soften your skin. Use daily until you see the desired effects.

2. Raw Potato

Potatoes have natural bleaching agents that can help you brighten up those circles. Take 1-2 cool potatoes and smash them until you can get the juice out. Now, dip a cotton ball in the potato juice and put on your (closed) eyes. Make sure the juice covers the black circles as well as the lids. Leave for 10-15 minutes and then rinse your eyelids well with cold water. If you don't want to use the juice, you can also just slice it like the cucumber with the same process, but the juice will be more potent.

3. Tomatoes

Yes, tomatoes too can help lighten the skin under your eyes. Take a spoon of tomato juice and mix with one spoon of lemon juice. Put the mix (using cotton balls again) gently on the eyes and leave for 10 minutes. Then, rinse with clean water. Do this twice a day to get rid of puffiness and dark circles.

4. Rose Water

A quick fix for those circles makes use of the great skin care benefits of rose water. Take cotton bandages and soak them in rose water for a few minutes. Then, place them on your closed eyelids for about 15 minutes. The rose water has a calming effect on the eyes and the skin around it. This solution can remove the dark circles completely if used twice a day for several weeks.

5. Almond Oil

Almond oil is another natural ingredient that benefits the delicate skin around our eyes. Regular use of almond oil can brighten the skin as well as nourish it. Take a little almond oil, place on the dark circles and gently massage it into the skin. Leave it overnight and wash with cold water in the morning. Do this every day until the circles are completely gone. If you don't have almond oil, you can also use a Vitamin E enriched oil.

6. Lemon Juice

The high vitamin C content in lemon juice can serve to remove the circles. Dip a cotton ball in fresh lemon juice and apply to the skin around your eyes for 10 minutes before washing it off. Another option is to make a thick mix by mixing one table spoon of lemon juice with 2 table spoons of tomato paste, a smidgen of humus flour and turmeric powder. Smear the mix gently around the eyes and leave on for 10-15 minutes, then wash with clean water. Repeat this 2-3 times a week and the skin will soon become much lighter.

7. Cold Water

Cold water can narrow the blood vessels underneath the eyes and help reduce puffiness and dark circles. Dip a clean, soft cloth in cold water or milk and put directly on the eyelids for several minutes Another option is to wrap a few ice cubes in a soft cloth and hold them under the eyes. A bag of frozen peas, of cold tea or even a cold spoon can also help. Repeat this 3-4 times a week for several weeks.

8. Apple

An apple too can provide a natural solution for removing those stubborn circles. Slice them up thickly and put under your eyes for 30 minutes before washing with cold water. Put some relaxing cream after this is done.Another course of action is to make a mash of green, cooked apples and put under the eyes for half an hour, then wash with lukewarm water.

9. Mint

Mint has a cooling effect on the skin that naturally removes the dark skin. Take a few fresh mint leaves and mash them gently. Smear the mix on your eyes and leave for 10-15 minutes. Gently rub away with a clean cloth. Another option is adding mint leaves to tomato juice and smearing under the eyes, leaving it for several minutes and then washing with cold water.

10. Cucumber

The cucumber is an age old solution for black circles. It is good at making your skin look lighter. For a quick fix for those circles, take a fresh cucumber and slice it into thick slices. Put them in the fridge for 30 minutes, then put the slices on the area of your eye for 10 minutes and rinse with water. This solution has a calming and refreshing effect.
Another option is to mix cucumber juice with lemon juice in equal amounts, and use a cotton ball to apply to the skin underneath the eyes. Leave the cotton on for about 15 minutes and then rinse with water. Do this every day for a week and the puffiness, as well as the dark areas, will shy away.

Ref: http://www.ba-bamail.com/

Home Remedies for Treating Varicose Veins

According to a number of studies, about 25 percent of all women and 10 percent of men are affected by varicose veins. Varicose veins are dilated and 'puffed up' veins that are usually in the legs that can be painful and have an unpleasant appearance. **But don't stop reading here, because there are a number of at-home remedies for treating varicose veins that could help you, or someone you know with the condition, avoid expensive and painful surgical procedures.** Varicose veins are usually genetic, so if someone in your family has had them, there is a greater chance that you will too. They are caused when the valves in the veins that push blood throughout your circulatory system weaken and become 'flappy', causing fluid to accumulate in the veins. The common signs for the development of varicose veins are tenderness around the area of an enlarged vein, swelling of the legs, a tightening or itching sensation in the legs and a feeling of heaviness in the legs.

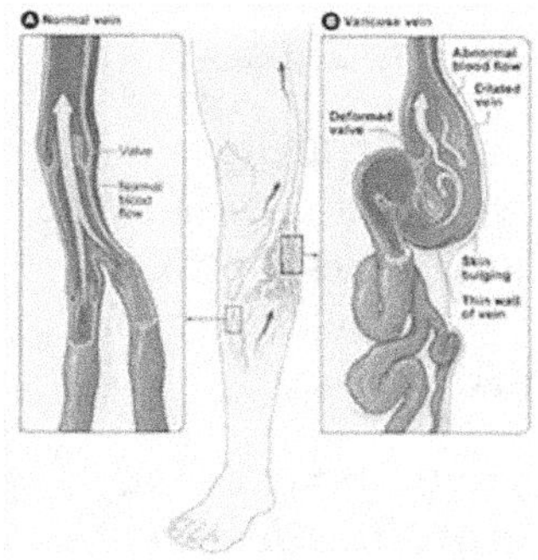

Although varicose veins are usually benign, meaning that they do not put your health at risk, their puffed up appearance is startling or discomforting for some, and therefore many doctors recommend cosmetic surgery to remove them. Yet these surgeries can be expensive and keep you off your feet, so it's best to try out some of these simple and completely natural remedies first.

1. Keep Your Feet Up

Just like on any long flight or an extended period sitting down, the blood rushes to your legs and causes them to feel heavy. The feeling with varicose veins is similar, and those that have the condition may experience swelling if they spend the day seated or on their feet. To remedy this uncomfortable feeling, it is best to recline with your legs elevated for anywhere up to an hour. This allows the blood to flow away from the legs and ankles and back towards the heart to decrease swelling and the feeling of heaviness.

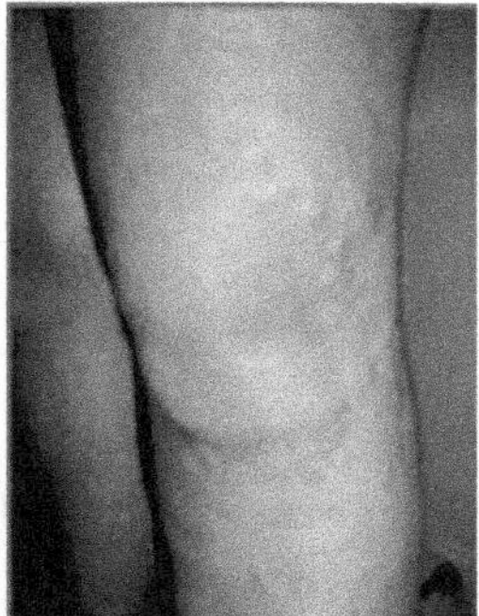

2. Ice Your Veins

Applying ice or a cold pack to your varicose veins can help minimize their appearance and reduce the swelling around the vein. This is because the application of cold restricts the bloodflow to the area of application, making the appearance of the swollen veins less apparent. It is also recommended to take a cold or lukewarm bath every so often to keep your bloodflow healthy and your veins and vessels working hard.

3. Exercise

Regularly performing cardiovascular exercise, either running, walking at a fast pace, biking or swimming, keeps your blood flowing as it should and prevents the pooling of liquids in your veins. It is recommended to perform at least 15 minutes of cardiovascular exercise every day (with approval from your doctor), and not just to stay fit. It has been shown that regular exercise can reduce the severity and appearance of varicose veins.

4. Flex Your Feet

Even if you aren't able to get in a full cardiovascular workout, doing a few leg raises or ankle circles will help keep your varicose veins in check. When you contract the muscles in your feet, the blood is forced upward out of your legs and towards the heart. By pointing and flexing your feet a few times, circling your ankles, or doing heel slips where you slide your heels back and forth can keep your circulation in check and blood out of your varicose veins.

5. Try A Compression Stocking

There are special compression socks and stockings that can be purchased at most pharmacies that will help improve circulation in your legs. As explained above, when pressure is applied to the lower legs, the blood is pushed up towards the heart and won't pool in your veins. You can get weaker compression stockings, 20mm Hg, or stronger ones at 60 mm Hg (the stronger versions usually require a prescription from a doctor). They come in a variety of colors and shapes for different parts of the leg and are usually comfortable enough (in the weak and mild versions) for everyday use.

If you or someone you know has varicose veins, you should consult your doctor to determine if you have a higher chance to experience clotting. These natural remedies will help mediate many of the effects of varicose veins, but there is no guarantee that they will completely disappear. There is no harm in trying!

Ref: http://www.ba-bamail.com/

A Guide to Relieving Gout Naturally

Gout is an arthritic health condition which affects the joints. This strongly genetic condition is more common in men than women, and to date has no known cure. This lifelong condition is caused by an excess amount of uric acid in the bloodstream, and attacks can be chronic.

Symptoms

- Crystals develop on the joints, followed by intense and sudden pain.
- Joints can swell, feel warm and tender, and can't bear the pressure of touch.
- You won't be able to move the affected joint much.
- Primarily felt in the feet, specifically the big toe, although it can flare up in the ankles, heels, knees, wrists, fingers or elbows.
- Skin surrounding the joint can turn red or purple, and appears bruised.
- After gout subsides you will have lingering discomfort around the joints and the skin around the joint will peel and feel itchy.
- After extended periods of gout, nodules may develop beneath the skin near the joints.
- Repeated bouts can also damage your joints and the kidney.
- Fluid sacs cushioning tissues around the elbow or knee may become inflamed.
- Symptoms often follow surgery or an illness.

Uric acid is caused by purines metabolizing, which are proteins found in organ meats, sardines, and anchovies, as well as alcohol. Some medication and supplements can also cause a buildup of uric acid. Examples include salicylates, the active component of aspirin, vitamin B3, too much vitamin C, and diuretics. Alcohol consumption, excess weight, and lead exposure can increase the chances of gout developing in those with a genetic susceptibility.

Doctors can recommend medicine to alleviate inflammation and pain, and usually opt for non-steroidal anti- inflammatory drugs (NSAIDs) such as ibuprofen and Tylenol. They can also prescribe medicine that work to lower uric acid levels and thereby lessen crystal formation, such as Colcrys, corticosteroids or allopurinol. Prescription medicine is often accompanied by strong side effects, and will require lifelong consumption. There are also several natural treatments which focus on relieving pain. The following 6 remedies' ingredients can easily be bought at the grocery store and can be administered in the comfort of your own home.

1. **Apple cider vinegar**

   This common cooking ingredient can raise your body's alkaline level, thereby reducing gout pain considerably. With its significant acidity, apple cider vinegar is commonly used to treat headaches and acid stomach. The best way to effectively ingest apple cider vinegar is by drinking it in a glass of water. Mix in one teaspoon to one glass of water and drink this mixture three times a day. To sweeten this bitter drink add some honey, which can also boost your body's anti-inflammatory response.

2. **Activated charcoal**

   One wouldn't naturally think of charcoal as a solution for any medical condition, but it seems activated charcoal is perfectly safe and it is known to absorb uric acid. The best way to use it to prevent gout flare-ups is by soaking in a bath of charcoal two to three times a week. You can add half a cup of charcoal powder to your bath water. When a paste is formed, add more water and soak your affected joint for at least half an hour. If you don't enjoy bathing, applying a charcoal paste directly to the skin of the affected joint. You can leave this on for half an hour and then remove with lukewarm water. The alternative solution is to consume activated charcoal tablets. This option does require consultation with your physician.

3. **Baking soda**

Baking soda is another household item that can be effective in treating gout pain. Baking soda reduces uric acid in the body. In an 8 oz. glass of water mix in half a teaspoon of baking soda and drink it. You can repeat this several times a day. No more than 4 teaspoons should be consumed in one day, and if you are over 60 years old, only 3 teaspoons per day should be consumed in total.
Note: This method is not recommended for anyone suffering from hypertension, as baking soda is known to elevate blood pressure.

4. **Cherries**

Cherries are another one of nature's treats that can help with gout. They are not only packed with antioxidants but also anthocyanins, which are known to reduce joint inflammation and can substantially reduce gout from flaring up in subsequent attacks. A daily serving of 15 to 20 cherries is recommended. If you want to avoid the high concentration of sugar in the fresh fruit, try drinking a glass of black cherry juice or a cherry juice concentrate daily.

5. **Apples**

The commonly heard phrase "an apple a day keeps the doctor away" can be especially true when it comes to gout. An apple after each meal, as endorsed by medical experts, can be very effective. The strong component of malic acid in apples can neutralize uric acid, thereby offering relief to both pain and inflammation. Some people don't enjoy the texture of apples – for those people I recommend trying apple juice or dicing the apples up and adding them to a bowl of cherries.

6. **Lemon juice**

Another way to neutralize excess uric acid in the blood stream, which can provide relief from pain caused by bouts of gout, is with lemon juice. The freshly squeezed juice of a lemon can alkalize the body. Another useful way to consume it is adding a lemon half to a glass of water, as this will be less strong than pure lemon juice. You can also mix the juice of a lemon with half a teaspoon of baking soda. When this mixture stops fizzing, add it to a glass of water and drink it immediately.

Source: top10homeremedies

Have You Tried Apple Cider Vinegar to Remove Skin Tags?

Skin tags are harmless, soft skin growths that tend to occur on the eyelids, neck, armpits, groin folds and under the breasts. They are most prone among middle-aged, obese adults. Removing a skin tag does not cause more to grow, and there is a harmless way to go about it, without having to make a trip to the doctor.

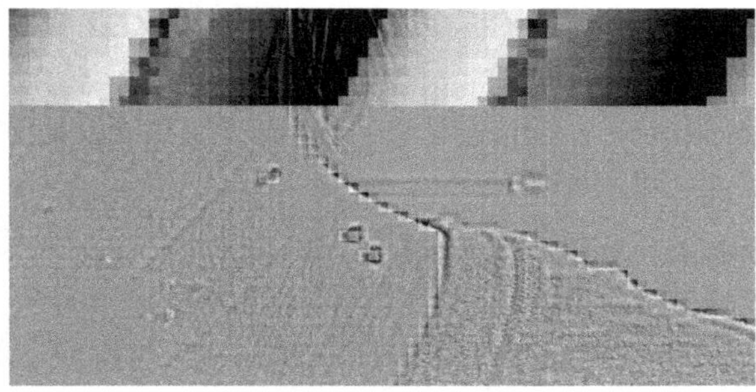

Instead of spending money on a cosmetic operation to safely remove skin tags, you should consider using a natural product as an alternative. As a result of its acidic properties, apple cider vinegar can be used to treat and help prevent a variety of common health problems. One of its benefits lies in its effectiveness in removing skin tags safely, and with minimal irritation to the surrounding area.

Why apple cider vinegar works

Apple cider vinegar doesn't attack the tag itself. Rather, it targets the tissue that causes and forms it. Once the tissue is destroyed, the tag turns black and falls off. Using apple cider vinegar targets the skin more deeply, ensuring that a tag is much less likely to grow again. Preferably, opt for an organically-produced bottle of apple cider vinegar, due to its higher quality.

Using apple cider vinegar to treat skin tags

The following detailed steps will ensure that you are performing the treatment correctly, effectively and safely:

Step 1: Clean the surrounding area well, washing it with warm water and soap. Dry it thoroughly. Ensure that all sweat and dirt is removed, as it may inhibit the apple cider vinegar from working effectively.

Step 2: Soak a small cotton ball in organic apple cider vinegar, squeezing out any excess vinegar before applying it to the skin tag.

Step 3: Once you have finished applying the cider vinegar to the skin tag, clean the area once again. Note that cider vinegar has a potent smell.

Step 4: Repeat the process for several days until you start to see results. At first, you will notice that the tag will darken in color, indicating that it will soon fall off completely.

Ref: http://www.ba-bamail.com/

How Can You Prevent Night Cramps?

Do you ever go to sleep in your cozy bed after a hard day and wake up with unexpected and painful leg cramps? This phenomenon is called Nocturnal Leg Cramps and Dr. Lisa Shives, from the Northshore Sleep Medicine in Illinois, says it's actually a very normal and common thing.

Nocturnal leg cramps are sudden, involuntary contractions that occur during the night or during times of rest. The cramping sensation may last a few seconds or minutes, but the pain from the cramps may linger for a much longer period. Nocturnal leg camps tend to happen to middle-aged or older populations, but people of any age can have them.

The exact cause of nocturnal leg cramps is not known. Some cases can occur without a triggering event, while others may be linked to prolonged sitting, dehydration or structural disorders. Research shows that about one third of the population above the age of 60 suffers from these cramps, with 6% reporting that it happens every night.

Here are some of the things that may cause this painful problem according to Dr. Shives:

- Medical conditions such as blood disease, diabetes, and muscle disorders.

- Changes in the hormone state due to pregnancy and hormone pills.

- A lack of calcium or a low ability to retain it in the body due to low levels of vitamin D.

- Weak and loose muscles that don't move during the day are more likely to cramp at night.

- Electrolyte imbalance caused by dehydration and not getting enough potassium and magnesium.

What can you do about it?

- Start by eating foods that have more potassium such as nuts, avocados, almonds and potatoes. Many people say that eating a banana before going to sleep prevents the cramps and the hard pains.

- Hot salt baths with Epsom salt for your feet will help relax your muscles and blood pressure.

- Get more exercises for your legs like evening walks and do some stretching before you go to sleep.

- Consider taking food supplements high on vitamin D, potassium and magnesium.

If none of these work and you still suffer from night cramps nearly every day then you should go see your doctor.

Good night!

Ref: http://www.ba-bamail.com/

How to Treat Excess Stomach Gas & Bloating

A large percentage of the population suffers from stomach gas from time to time, yet it is rarely discussed, usually because we're too embarrassed to say we're gassy. But folks, we all are sometimes, and there's absolutely no reason to be ashamed of it. It is a very uncomfortable feeling, and can cause real pain.

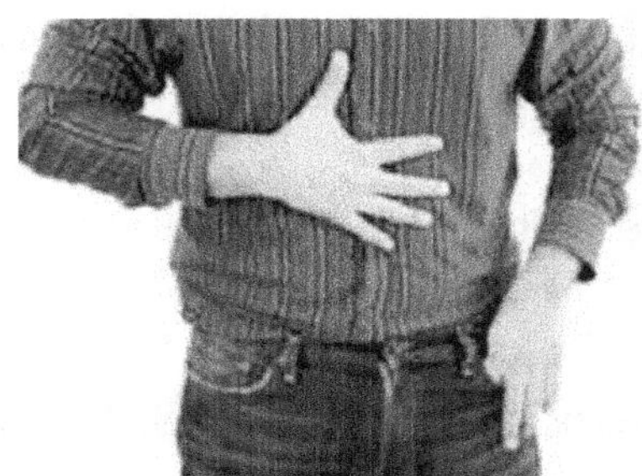

This is a problem that is becoming more prevalent due to modern food groups which encourage the build-up of gas in our system. But there are easy ways to fix this in your own home.

Causes of stomach gas build-up

~ Gas is mainly formed due to small fragmented stool as a result of eating refined diet lacking in vegetable fibre. These fragmented stool remain in the colon for too long, allowing colonic bacteria to ferment it. If one takes a high fibre diet it produce bulky stool that evacuates completely and so very little gas is formed.

~ Intolerance to certain types of food can also cause this effect.

~ Constipation will often lead to excess gas.

Symptoms of stomach gas:

- Frequent passing of gas

- Feeling as if bloated

- Loss of appetite

- Abdomen feels 'tight'

- Belching

- Jabbing chest pain

Getting rid of the excess stomach gas

1. **Lie Down or try different positions**
   Lie down and keep your head elevated, this position will help pass the discomfort you are feeling in a few minutes. Remain in this position until the discomfort you're feeling is gone. You can lie down on your side, but still keep your head elevated. If you are in distress, you can try to curl up so your head is touching the floor and your rear is in the air, this will encourage the passing of gas from your system.
   When you are trying to push the gas out of your abdomen, make sure to do so on an empty stomach or over a toilet.

2. **Drink more**
   Having excess gas in your stomach is usually a sign of poor digestion, drinking plenty of fluid helps move the undigested remnants of the food from the colon. This is especially true if you've eaten a lot of fiber rich foods, which encourage undigested food particles to accumulate in the colon. So drink up.
   Hot liquids help the most, try herbal tea, but even coffee will help get that gas moving.

3. **Add mustard**
   Mustard is said to decrease the amount of gas in the body as well as preventing its build-up, so try and add it to one of your daily meals.

4. **Baking Soda**
   Add a spoonful of baking soda to a cup of hot water and mix well. Drink this every couple of hours for quick relief.

5. **Add Indian spices**
   Turmeric, cumin and cardamom are known to aid good digestion.

6. **Add ginger**
   Adding ginger to your food or chewing on the root will offer quick relief and aid your digestion.

7. **Certain fruit can help**
   Drink lemon juice or other citrus fruit juices. The papaya is a wonderful fruit to eat when bloated, and is one of the best means for getting rid of gas quickly.

8. **Avoid carbonated drinks**
   Consuming carbonated drinks is a big no no if you want to decrease the amount of gas in the body. Drinking these will lead to an increase in gas and may also lead to chest pain

Ref: http://www.ba-bamail.com/

Neuropathy Causes and Natural Solutions

The term **Neuropathy** is short for *'peripheral neuropathy'*. It relates to nerve damage suffered by the peripheral nervous system, which is in charge of our nerves outside the brain and spinal cord. Neuropathy is a complication that can be caused by a number of various conditions. Physical trauma, repetitive injury, infections, metabolic problems and exposure to toxins and some drugs can all lead to peripheral neuropathy.

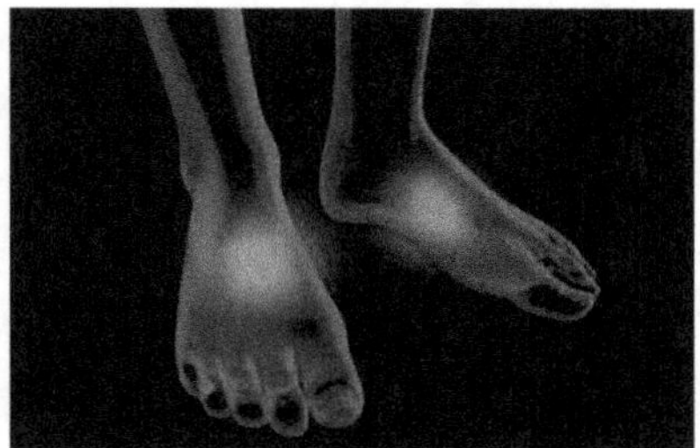

Signs and symptoms of neuropathy

Neuropathy usually starts as a tingling or burning sensation at our extremities, such as fingers and toes. There is also a loss of sensation at the edge of the nerves that patients have reported feeling like they are wearing a thin stocking or glove on their hands.

The precise symptoms differ from patient to patient based on the types of nerves affected. There are three types of nerves that may be affected by neuropathy: sensory, motor and autonomic.

Sensory nerves

Sensory nerves are responsible for collecting sensory information for the body, such as touch. Neuropathy of the sensory nerves can be expressed as:

- Spreading numbness and tingling in hands and/or feet (which can spread to the arms and legs).

- Burning, sharp or electric-like pain

- Extreme sensitivity to touch

- Problems with coordination

Motor nerves:

Motor nerves are the nerves responsible for activating our muscles and control movements.

- Muscle weakness

- Paralysis

Autonomic nerves:

Autonomic nerves are responsible for internal actions of the body, such as regulating digestion, heat and blood pressure.

- Intolerance to heat

- Problems with digestion, bladder and bowel control

- Dizziness (or lightheadedness) brought about by problems with blood pressure.

A common cause of neuropathy: Diabetes

For diabetics, neuropathy can be quite common. That said, about 50% of diabetics who have neuropathy won't notice the symptoms, and it will stay on a very low level. For the other 50%, however, the symptoms will be unavoidable. Pain is the most common complaint, usually a 'prickling', 'stabbing' or 'burning' pain, that happens mostly at night. This, along with a numbness that feels as if the limb is 'asleep' - occurs predominantly in the toes, feet and legs.

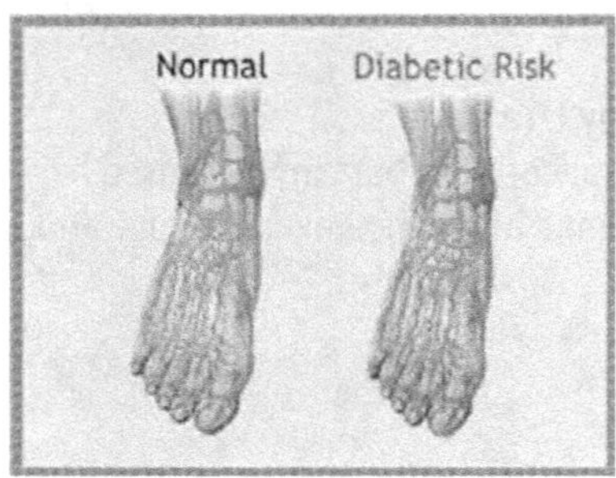

What do doctors prescribe for this condition?

Most doctors will stick to the old medical regime of anti-depressants, anti-convulsants, steroid and cortisone injections, lidocaine patches and pain killers. These are powerful drugs that address the

painful sensations for short and long term relief. However, as powerful drugs, they have a host of side-effects and must be administered very carefully. Some medical practitioners recommend electrical stimulation of the pain area and of the spine. The medical community is united in agreement that more solutions to this problem are required, but progress has been very slow from the medical and drug industry so far.

Natural solutions to neuropathy

First off, if you are suffering from diabetes related neuropathy, you must do the following:

- Give up smoking

- Cut down on alcohol consumption or give it up altogether

- Maintain a healthy weight

- Exercise

Other recommended habits for those suffering from neuropathy include: Wearing clothing that causes less irritation, such as cotton, covering the sensitive areas with wound dressing or cling film and using cold packs. Stress relief is also a big help when it comes to neuropathy, and so relaxation techniques are a big help, such as yoga, meditation and acupuncture.

Vitamin therapy

Clinical studies have shown that certain supplements can have a cumulative effect on the symptoms and causes of neuropathy. These herbal extracts can be taken without worry that they may clash with a parallel medical treatment. Certain herbal extracts and formulas offer a level of relief that has rarely been reached by just using medical procedures. This must be taken daily to achieve the desired relief.

Vitamins B1, B2, B6 and B12.

Vitamin B deficiency is one of the major causes of neuropathy, and also one of the best natural solutions. All herbal extracts contain large amounts of vitamin B1, usually in its common form of thiamine. Recent natural medications have reverted to using benfotiamine, which has been found to be significantly more effective in delivering vitamin B than thiamine is (x3).

Stabilized R-Alpha Lipoic Acid (R-ALA)

This powerful antioxidant that is one of the few, rare materials that can pass through the brain's blood/brain barrier to enter the brain and go directly where it is needed the most.

Most importantly, it has a specific effect on the nerves that eases the pain and numbness associated with neuropathy, and promotes better blood flow and oxygen to the nerves.
Recent studies have reported that just by using the R-ALA alone, orally, has reduced symptoms of europathy.

Neuropathy support formulas

These days, it is common for those suffering from neuropathy to take both medical and vitamin therapies, combining short-term treatment with the cumulative effects of correct nutrition.

The best formulas (so make sure they have these in the ingredient list) include vitamins B1, B2 and B12, as well as Vitamin D, R-ALA and materials that relax your nervous system, avoiding overstimulation.

I personally recommend checking those out for anyone who is really looking for a solution to their neuropathy problem, or is worried they are developing one. For diabetes patients, this would be a good way to perhaps prevent the onset of neuropathic symptoms.

Ref: http://www.ba-bamail.com/

Overcoming the Symptoms of Adrenal Fatigue Syndrome

Adrenal fatigue is a much more common problem than you might think. If you've been feeling extremely tired lately, you could have adrenal fatigue syndrome, which is also called adrenal insufficiency.

This affliction occurs because of the adrenal gland malfunctioning. About 80% of the world's population is thought to experience it at some point.

Adrenal fatigue can hinder you when you're doing housework or at your job, however, the good news is that it's easy to overcome. The most important step is to have adrenal fatigue diagnosed, and that starts with acknowledging any symptoms our may have.

The Most Common Signs

One of the biggest red flags for adrenal fatigue is getting a good night's sleep and waking up more tired than when you went to bed. This tends to be the first thing that people with adrenal fatigue notice about themselves.

If it seems to be occurring to you repeatedly, then you definitely shouldn't overlook it.

The second most prevalent symptom of adrenal fatigue is anxiety. Feeling extremely overwhelmed by everything going on around you can be put down to adrenal fatigue or what's known as "burnout syndrome", which you get from overwork and not resting enough.

Anxiety caused by adrenal fatigue is usually accompanied by poor memory and an inability to focus or concentrate.

If you're seemingly unable to lose weight, it might also indicate that your adrenal gland isn't working properly. This is especially true if you've lowered your calorie intake and are working out regularly.

How to Overcome It

If you're experiencing the symptoms outlined above, the first thing you need to do is cut all the stimulants and irritants out of your diet, with specific reference to caffeine and sugar.

Next, you need to increase your magnesium and vitamin B complex intake, as these two essential nutrients will stimulate your adrenal glands and balance your blood sugar levels.

In addition to the nutrients above, you should also increase your daily intake of healthy amino acids, such as Omega 3 and Omega 6. You can do this by adding olive oil to your salads – it's a great source of amino acids. Try combining extra virgin olive oil with dark, leafy greens such as chard, kale or spinach. You can also try seaweed, as it is particularly rich in minerals.

Also consider taking natural dietary supplements containing adaptogenic herbal extracts, roots and natural plants such as ginseng, rhodiola, ashwagandha and holy basil. Note that there's only so much that these supplements can do, so take them in conjunction with B vitamins, selenium and vitamin D.

Vitamin D helps relieve stress, allowing you to get a better night's sleep. It works best in combination with selenium and magnesium, which improve adrenal gland function.

If your day-to-day life is stressful, see what you can do to reduce it. Try yoga, breathing exercises, melotherapy or aromatherapy.

Exercise is always good for keep stress levels down – jogging, swimming, hiking or even walking for half an hour each day can help you keep them manageable.

Conclusion

You don't need to let adrenal insufficiency wreak havoc on your life.

Remember to do the following:

- Get rid of caffeine
- Eat more fruit and vegetables
- Stay hydrated
- Cut down on sugar and empty calories
- Remove fast food from your diet
- Exercise to keep stress levels down
- Live by these rules and you'll remain healthy, happy and energetic for many years to come!

Content Source: Natural Solution Today

8 Pressure Points That Reduce Stress

We all have our ways of dealing with stress. Some people escape to a sunny beach, some prefer a nice glass of wine, and others even do their best to ignore it. Each way has its advantages (and sometimes disadvantages), but we can't always do what helps at the exact moment we need to. This is where pressure points become a quick and effective long-term solution. Pressure points are areas in the body that can trigger various effects in our bodies and minds when pressure is applied to them.

The Scalp

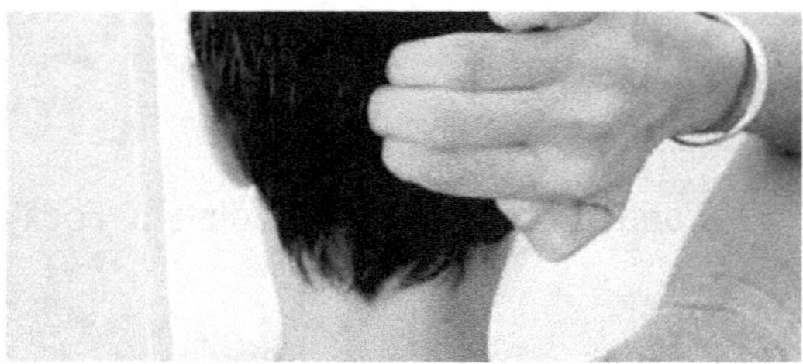

The Scalp is full of pressure points, many that can effectively and discretely reduce stress levels. You can sit at your office desk, lean back and use two fingers to massage the point where the neck meets the skull for about 20 seconds. Much of the stress we accumulate during the day collects in the shoulders and neck muscles, and applying pressure to this point can relieve much of it.

The Ear

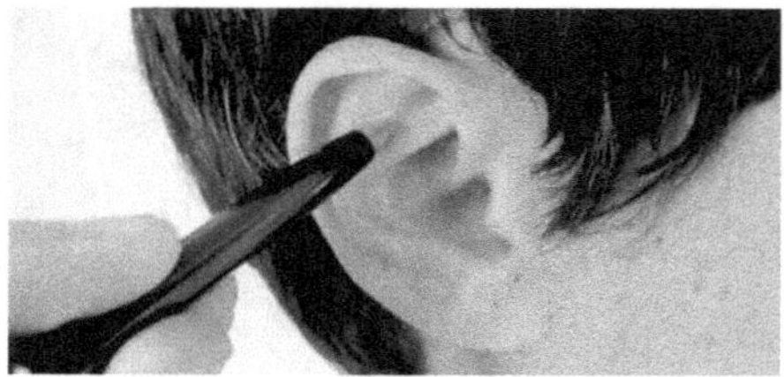

This pressure point is known as *Shen Men* (The Spirit Gate), and some experts claim it's the best stress-relieving point in the body. In reflexology, it's also used to reduce inflammation and pain throughout the body. It's recommended that you massage this spot with a cotton bud or even a pen, and to take deep, slow breaths during the massage.

The Chest

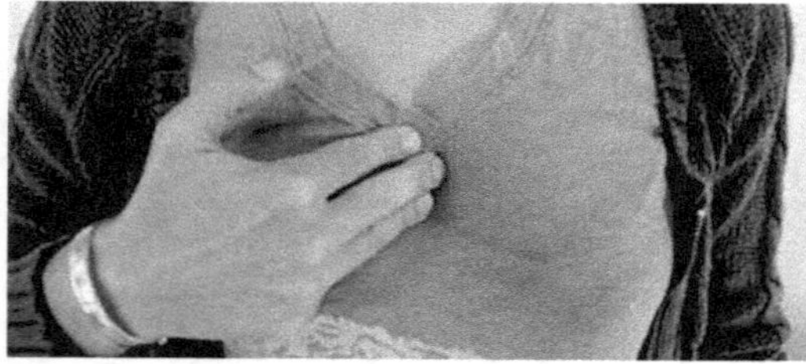

Like

Stress can make us forget to breathe, or take shallow breaths. This point helps reduce the stress that accumulates in your chest, while reminding you to breathe normally again. Use three fingers to massage this point, or one finger to tap rhythmically on the area while taking deep breaths. If you experience chronic stress, combine massaging this point with the point between your eyebrows. The connection between these two points helps to calm the nervous system.

The Stomach Like

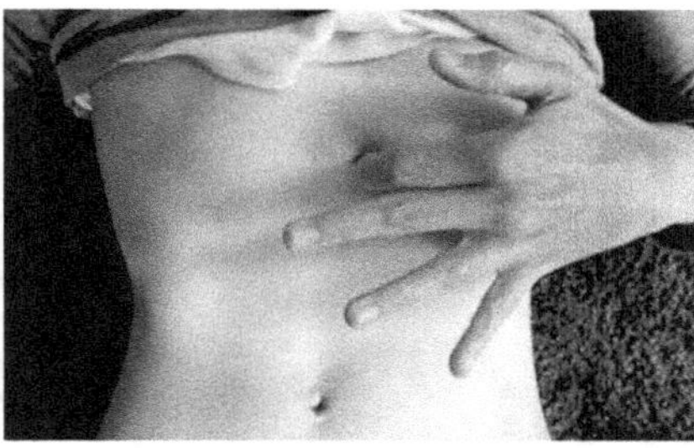

Many reflexologists prefer to use this point because it helps create movement that frees the chest and diaphragm, which improves the breathing process. Patients who have this treatment instinctively take deeper breaths and almost always report a sensation or relief.

The Forearm

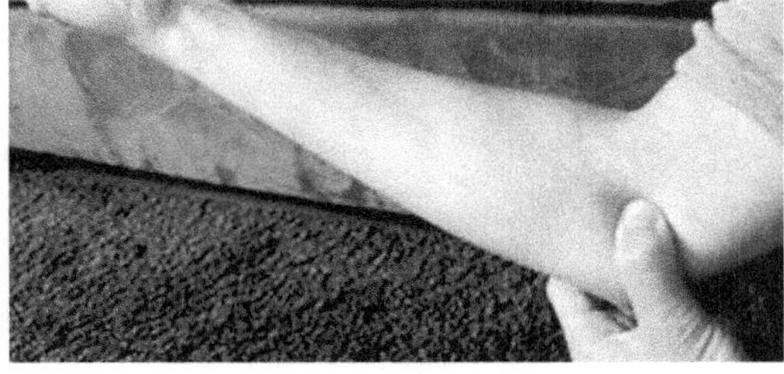

This is a classic spot for reflexology and acupuncture. Stress and anxiety create reverse energy flow in the body, which this spot is supposed to repair. It helps your energy to move in the right direction while aiding your mental focus and reducing stress.

The Palm

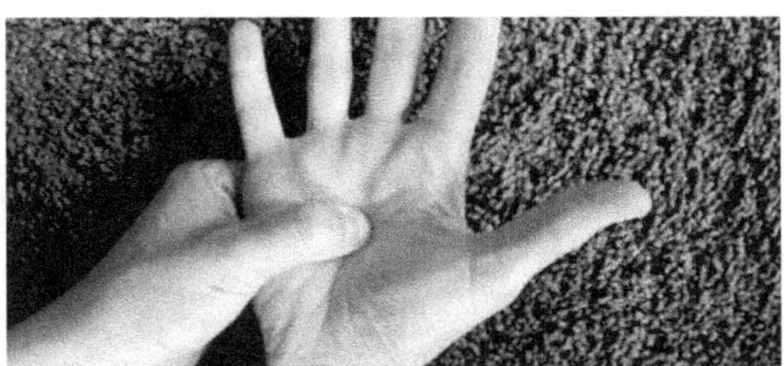

The moment you press on this spot, you'll feel your stress evaporating. It is located on one of the most important meridians (an energy channel), which affects the heart, liver, and pancreas. It is believed that much of the stress we experience is stored in the liver, so applying pressure on this point is highly effective. It is also a great spot for treating headaches, stomachaches, indigestion, and insomnia — all of which could be symptoms of stress.

The Calves

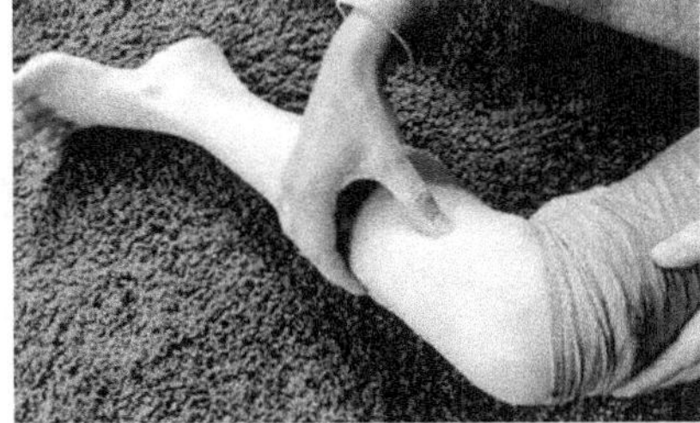

Like

If you feel stress in the upper part of your body, massaging this spot is perfect. The area could be quite tender in people who deal with a lot of stress, and in women in particular.

The Foot

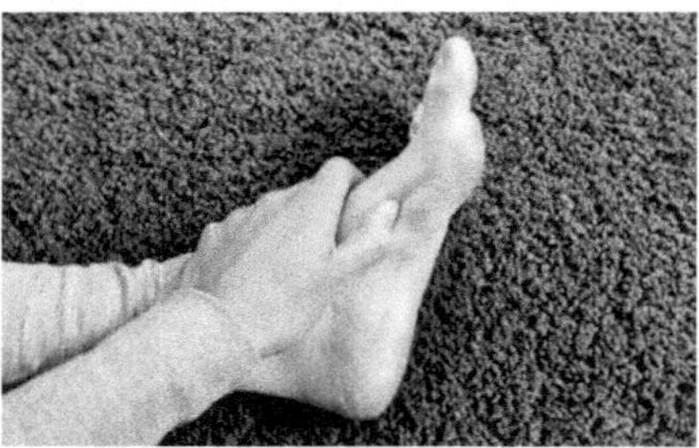

Pressure on this point can help ease a stressed mind that keeps rethinking whatever it is that causes your stress. Some reflexologists believe that this is the best meridian for treating the pancreas and that its location, in the center of the foot, helps patients reduce stress and provide better attention to their bodies

Ref: http://www.ba-bamail.com/

5 Methods to Help You Get Rid of a Dry Cough

A persistent dry cough can be irritating to handle. The good news is that there are a number of remedies you can try to reduce or eliminate your cough. On this note, it is important to bear in mind that if your cough persists for more than three weeks, you should consult with your doctor. Meanwhile, here are some methods I have found to work on me:

1. **Stay Hydrated**

   Keep your throat moist: A postnasal drip may be a reason for your cough. This occurs when drainage from your nose drips into the back of your throat, which usually happens after a cold or the flu. Staying hydrated and drinking plenty of fluids can thin out the mucus caused by colds.

   Gargle warm salt water: To help relieve the pain in your throat and reduce inflammation, try gargling some warm salt water before going to bed.

   Drink plenty of warm water: Warm water rehydrates the throat better than hot water - which can cause irritation. Opt for warm tea, such as aniseed, to help you stay hydrated. It will help soothe your throat and reduce a cough. Add cinnamon to gain extra relief.

   Boil ginger with your tea leaves: Use ginger to naturally unblock a congested nose and chest. Spice it up with a dash of pepper and add several basil leaves to relieve congestion.

   Drink hot cinnamon with honey and milk before bed: Cinnamon and honey are a great combination to help fight infection, decrease swelling or provide antioxidant properties to help cure a sore throat. Combine 1/2 teaspoon cinnamon and 1 tablespoon sugar in a saucepan. Add 1/8 teaspoon baking soda and 8 ounces milk, mixing thoroughly. Heat until it begins to simmer, but do not boil. Allow to cool and add 1 tablespoon honey, stirring until the honey dissolves completely. Drink while warm.

   Drink pineapple juice: Pineapples are beneficial for your health, especially for a cough. In fact according to a study conducted in 2010, pineapple juice is 5 times more effective than cough syrup. The juice softens the larynx and does not leave any residue which may cause you to cough more. It is also a better alternative to orange or lemon juice. Grape juice is also good to opt for when you have a cough. To add to the benefits, mix one teaspoon of honey in a cup of grape juice.

   Drink some oregano tea: Simply boil a tablespoon of oregano leaves in a cup of water. Once the water has boiled, strain the oregano out and enjoy.

2. **Consume Soothing Food**

   Soothe your throat with honey: The health benefits of honey are incredible. In soothing a sore throat, honey will help moisten your tonsils, reducing throat irritation. Rose petal infused water is also a good alternative, as the rose essence helps break up the mucus.

   Use essential oils: Essential oils can be used for a variety of ailments. The following essential oils may be useful in reducing a persistent cough: eucalyptus, peppermint, rosemary, sage, tea tree, sandalwood, cedarwood, frankincense and hyssop. Whichever you choose, add 1 to 2 drops of the essential oil to your hands, rubbing them together and cupping them over your nose. Take 4 to 6 deep breaths.

   Make a homemade cough syrup: Try an herbal cough syrup by mixing two ounces of the herb mixture to one quart of water. Try fennel, licorice, slippery elm bark, cinnamon, ginger root and orange peel. Simmer the herbs in water, until the mixture is reduced by half, then strain and add one cup of honey, stirring until thoroughly mixed.

   Eat warm chicken soup: The steam from the soup will help open the upper respiratory membranes, while the warmth will help soothe your throat. Chicken is packed with protein, and will therefore help you keep your strength. Try these chicken soup recipes to help fight a cough.

3. **Use a Humidifier and Steam to Your Advantage**

   The benefits of using a humidifier: Dry air can cause secretions in your nose to dry up, leading to a cough. A humidifier can help. Be cautious though, as using it too much (if not cleaned properly) can pump fungus and mold back into the air, prolonging your cough.

   Take a steamy hot shower: Turn off the fan and close all the windows, creating your very own steam room in the bathroom. Steam is an excellent remedy for coughs caused by colds, allergies and asthma as it helps loosen secretions in your nose.

Inhale steam from a boiling pot of water: Boil a pot of water. Once boiled, remove from the stovetop, and place it on a heat-proof surface. Lean over the water, placing a towel over your head and breathe in the steam. Add some thyme leaves to the water for extra relief.

4. Take Medication to Speed up Recovery

Use a decongestant: If your cough is caused by postnasal drip, consider taking a decongestant, which shrinks nasal tissue that has become swollen, reducing mucus.

Take an antihistamine: This type of medication is especially effective during allergy season, or if your cough is an allergic reaction to something in your environment, such as pets or mold.

5. Treat the Underlying Problem

Visit your doctor to diagnose an infection: Your cough may be a result of a bacterial infection. In which case, visit your doctor to prescribe antibiotics.

Check your environment for irritants: Your cough could be caused by sinus irritation, from a new perfume or spray. Smoke is also a serious cause of coughing and may play a factor.

Stomach irritation may be a cause: If you suffer from GERD (a chronic digestive disease) or frequent heartburn, take steps to minimize their effects. Avoid lying down three hours after meals and avoid spicy food or other food that may trigger your symptoms.

Check your medication: Some medications, particularly ACE inhibitors may cause a chronic cough. If the medication you are using leads to such an effect, discuss different options of medication with your doctor.

Avoid dust and other allergens: Thorough cleaning or air filters can remove dust and allergens from your environment. If this is not possible, use allergy medication to treat a chronic cough.

Ref: http://www.ba-bamail.com/

A Guide to Relieving Gout Naturally

Gout is an arthritic health condition which affects the joints. This strongly genetic condition is more common in men than women, and to date has no known cure. This lifelong condition is caused by an excess amount of uric acid in the bloodstream, and attacks can be chronic.

Symptoms

- Crystals develop on the joints, followed by intense and sudden pain.
- Joints can swell, feel warm and tender, and can't bear the pressure of touch.
- You won't be able to move the affected joint much.
- Primarily felt in the feet, specifically the big toe, although it can flare up in the ankles, heels, knees, wrists, fingers or elbows.
- Skin surrounding the joint can turn red or purple, and appears bruised.
- After gout subsides you will have lingering discomfort around the joints and the skin around the joint will peel and feel itchy.
- After extended periods of gout, nodules may develop beneath the skin near the joints.
- Repeated bouts can also damage your joints and the kidney.
- Fluid sacs cushioning tissues around the elbow or knee may become inflamed.
- Symptoms often follow surgery or an illness.

Uric acid is caused by purines metabolizing, which are proteins found in organ meats, sardines, and anchovies, as well as alcohol. Some medication and supplements can also cause a buildup of uric acid. Examples include salicylates, the active component of aspirin, vitamin B3, too much vitamin C, and diuretics. Alcohol consumption, excess weight, and lead exposure can increase the chances of gout developing in those with a genetic susceptibility. Doctors can recommend medicine to alleviate inflammation and pain, and usually opt for non-steroidal anti- inflammatory drugs (NSAIDs) such as ibuprofen and Tylenol. They can also prescribe medicine that work to lower uric acid levels and thereby lessen crystal formation, such as Colcrys, corticosteroids or allopurinol. Prescription medicine is often accompanied by strong side effects, and will require lifelong consumption. There are also several natural treatments which focus on relieving pain. The following 6 remedies' ingredients can easily be bought at the grocery store and can be administered in the comfort of your own home.

1. Apple cider vinegar

This common cooking ingredient can raise your body's alkaline level, thereby reducing gout pain considerably. With its significant acidity, apple cider vinegar is commonly used to treat headaches and acid stomach. The best way to effectively ingest apple cider vinegar is by drinking it in a glass of water. Mix in one teaspoon to one glass of water and drink this mixture three times a day. To sweeten this bitter drink add some honey, which can also boost your body's anti-inflammatory response.

2. Activated charcoal

One wouldn't naturally think of charcoal as a solution for any medical condition, but it seems activated charcoal is perfectly safe and it is known to absorb uric acid. The best way to use it to prevent gout flare-ups is by soaking in a bath of charcoal two to three times a week. You can add half a cup of charcoal powder to your bath water. When a paste is formed, add more water and soak your affected joint for at least half an hour.

If you don't enjoy bathing, applying a charcoal paste directly to the skin of the affected joint. You can leave this on for half an hour and then remove with lukewarm water. The alternative solution is to consume activated charcoal tablets. This option does require consultation with your physician.

3. **Baking soda**

Baking soda is another household item that can be effective in treating gout pain. Baking soda reduces uric acid in the body. In an 8 oz. glass of water mix in half a teaspoon of baking soda and drink it. You can repeat this several times a day. No more than 4 teaspoons should be consumed in one day, and if you are over 60 years old, only 3 teaspoons per day should be consumed in total.
Note: This method is not recommended for anyone suffering from hypertension, as baking soda is known to elevate blood pressure.

4. **Cherries**

Cherries are another one of nature's treats that can help with gout. They are not only packed with antioxidants but also anthocyanins, which are known to reduce joint inflammation and can substantially reduce gout from flaring up in subsequent attacks. A daily serving of 15 to 20 cherries is recommended. If you want to avoid the high concentration of sugar in the fresh fruit, try drinking a glass of black cherry juice or a cherry juice concentrate daily.

5. **Apples**

The commonly heard phrase "an apple a day keeps the doctor away" can be especially true when it comes to gout. An apple after each meal, as endorsed by medical experts, can be very effective. The strong component of malic acid in apples can neutralize uric acid, thereby offering relief to both pain and inflammation. Some people don't enjoy the texture of apples – for those people I recommend trying apple juice or dicing the apples up and adding them to a bowl of cherries.

6. **Lemon juice**

Another way to neutralize excess uric acid in the blood stream, which can provide relief from pain caused by bouts of gout, is with lemon juice. The freshly squeezed juice of a lemon can alkalize the body. Another useful way to consume it is adding a lemon half to a glass of water, as this will be less strong than pure lemon juice. You can also mix the juice of a lemon with half a teaspoon of baking soda. When this mixture stops fizzing, add it to a glass of water and drink it immediately.

Ref: Source: top10homeremedies

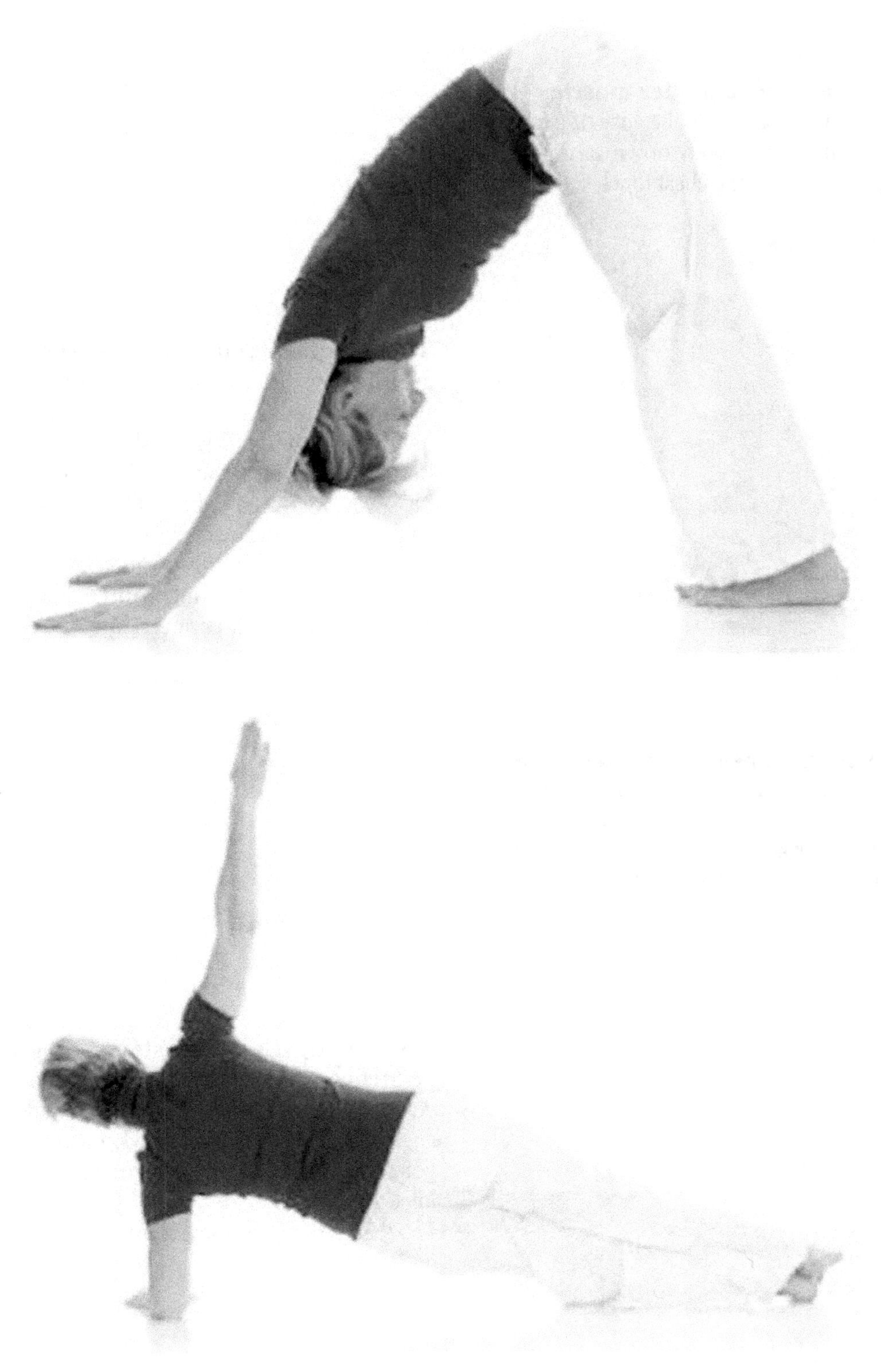

7 Easy Home Exercises to Keep You Healthy

Modern living has made many things easier for us. Unfortunately, it also has the side-effect of making our lives more sedentary and us - downright lazy. That is why it's more important than ever to work the body a little when we get the chance, whether we're at home or at work. A little use of muscles will keep your aches down, prevent muscular diseases and your chances of contracting cardiovascular diseases or blood clots. We highly recommend taking the time to perform these 7 simple exercises, which can be done almost anywhere.

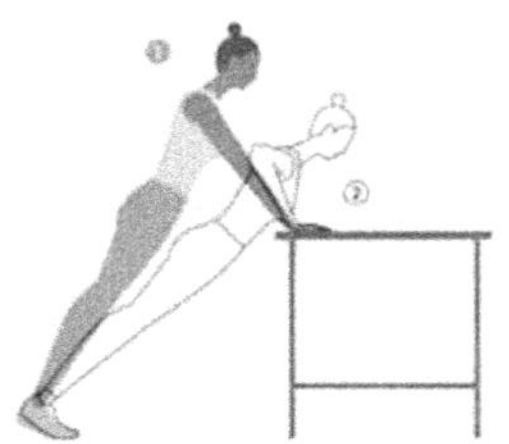

To strengthen the chest and shoulder muscles - push-ups at an incline: Put your palms on the edge of a table and straighten your elbows. Bend your body downward until the elbows are at 90 degree angles, or the chest touches the table, and go back up.
Do 3 sets of 20 repetitions.

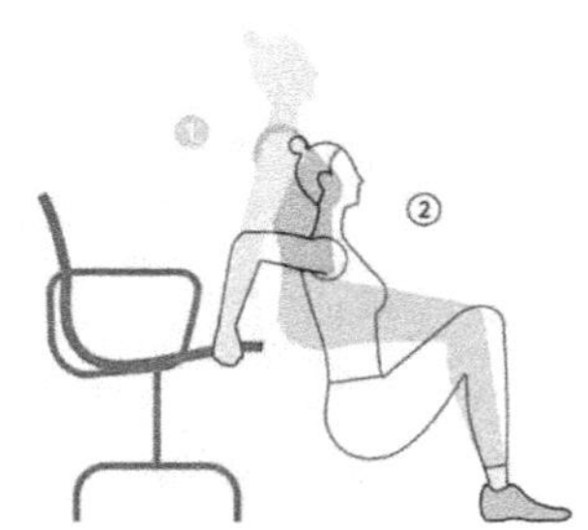

To strengthen your triceps -reverse elbow bends: To get into the position you'll need to sit at the edge of a chair (without wheels and against a wall to prevent falling) with your hands holding its sides, and slowly move forward with your buttocks until only your hands are supporting your sitting. Now you are in the right position to begin the exercise. Bend your mid section down towards the floor until your elbows are at 90 degrees. Stay in this position about 1 second and then go slowly back to the starting point.
Do 3 sets of 10-15 repetitions.

To strengthen the quadriceps thigh muscles - one legged squat: Stand straight on one leg facing forwards, and bend the leg slowly to a sitting position until your rear is almost at a 90 degree angle to your legs. Keep your weight focused on the leg you're standing on. Repeat this 10 times for each leg - for 3 sets.

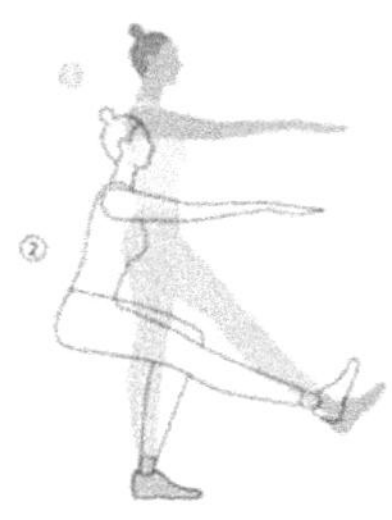

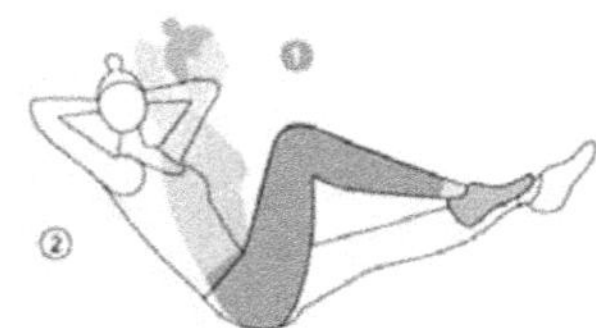

To strengthen the stomach muscles Bicycle crunches: Start at a sitting position with your hands behind your head, the legs in the air and the knees at a 90 degree angle. Do a sit up as you slowly move your right elbow to your left knee, and then your left elbow to your right knee.
Do 3 sets of 20 repetitions.

To strengthen the Biceps - Isometric practice: Sit at a table with your hands underneath it. Using your biceps, try and raise your hands up, with the elbows pressed against your body, for 10-20 seconds, then release. Repeat 5 times.
Do 3 sets of 5 repetitions.

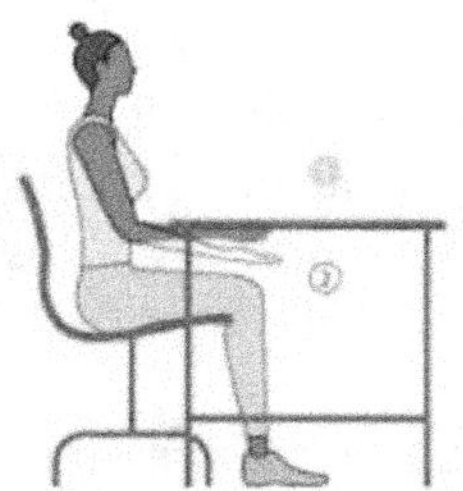

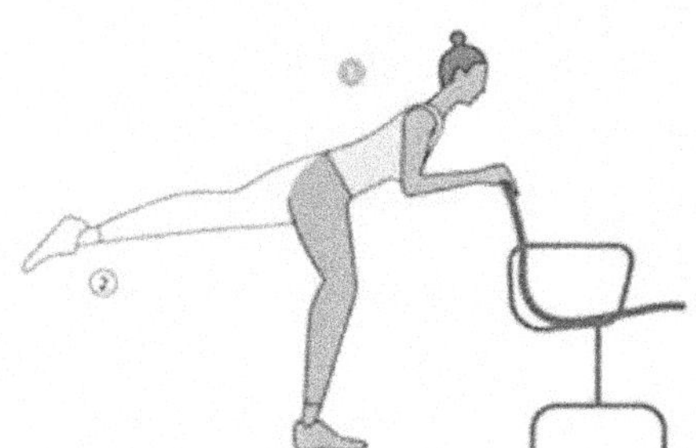

To strengthen the posterior thigh muscles and back - Donkey kicks: Stand with your legs slightly bent as you are holding on to a chair back. Hold your stomach in while you lift your right leg for a slow kick, until parallel to the floor.
Do 3 sets of 20 repetitions

To strengthen your stomach muscles - Sitting knee bends: Sit on a chair with your rear on the edge of it. Lay back at an angle of 45 degree and support your stance with your elbows resting on the arm rests, and bring up your knees in the direction of the body. Now, straighten your knees until your legs are parallel to the floor.
Do 3 sets of 20 repetitions.

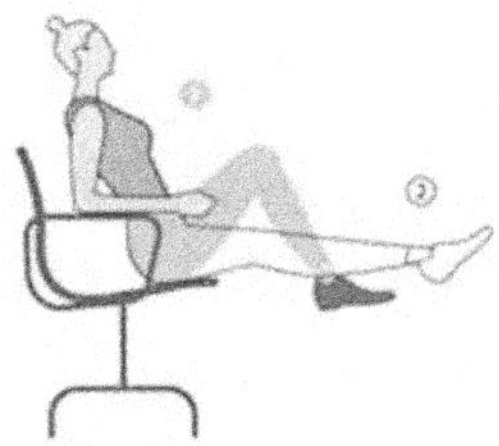

7 Exercises That'll Improve Eye Health

Other than our heart, our eye muscles are the hardest working muscle group in the body. It doesn't matter whether you're at work, at the gym or relaxing at home – we still stare at screens. These habits weaken our eye muscles, making them tired and less efficient, which in turn weakens our eyesight and exacerbates existing problems. These six easy exercises will reduce the strain on your eyes – a leading cause of tension and tiredness.

Important: Take a 20-second break between each set.

1. **Focusing on Different Distances**
    This exercise works on the inner eye muscles.

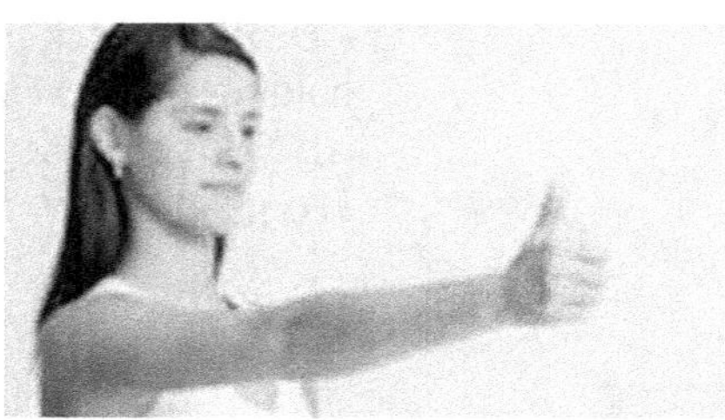

Repetitions: 5
Sets: 3

- Stand or sit comfortably.
- Place your thumb approximately 10 inches away from your face and focus on it.
- Take a deep breath and focus on an object that's 10-20ft away.
- Repeat by changing focus between objects with every deep breath.

2. **Stretching the Medial and Lateral Eye Muscles**
    This exercise will stretch and strengthen the muscles that control the eye's horizontal and vertical movement.

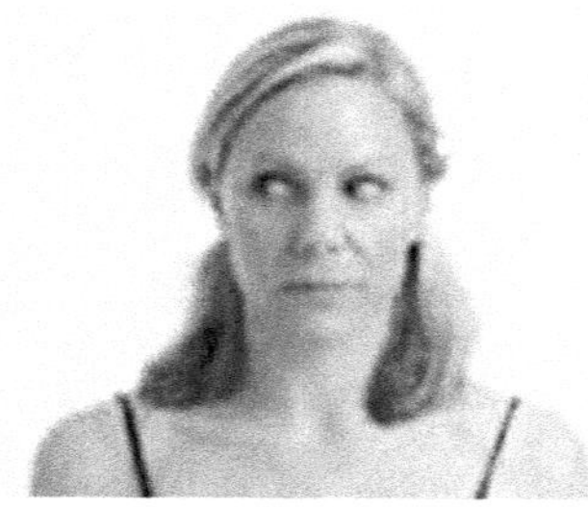

Repetitions: 3
Sets: 3

- Sit comfortably while maintaining an upright position.
- Look at the leftmost point you can without moving your head. Focus on this point for 5 seconds.
- Blink a few times and return the eye to its normal resting state.
- Look at the rightmost point you can without moving your head. Focus on that point for 5 seconds.
- Blink a few times and return the eye to its normal resting state.
- Repeat the exercise by looking at the upper-most/lowest point. Remember to blink between each stretch.

3. **Relaxing the Eyes**
    This exercise will reduce tension and stress around the eyes and is recommended when taking a break from working on the computer.

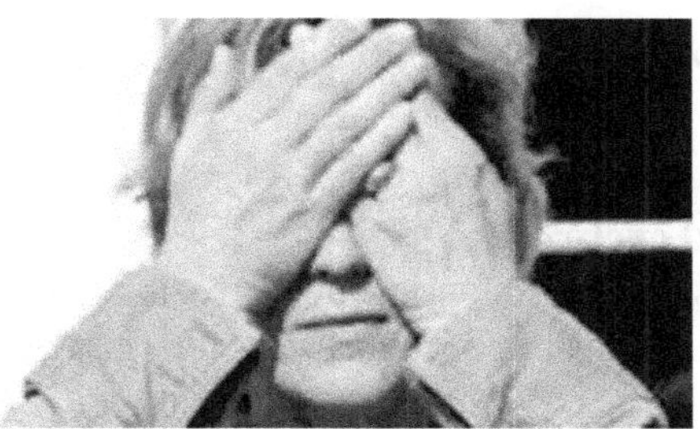

Duration: 5-10 minutes

- Sit comfortably and take a few deep breaths.
- Lean your elbows on a desk (place a pillow underneath to reduce strain on the elbows).
- Rub your palms together to warm them up.
- Close your eyes and cover them with your palms. Your fingers should be on your forehead, and the bottom of your palms should lean on your cheekbones.
- Make sure not to put pressure on your eyes by pressing your palms on them. To be sure, try blinking.
- Remain in this state for 5-10 minutes (it's recommended that you use a timer).
- If your eyes still feel tired, repeat it.

4. **Half-Closing Your Eyes**
This exercise, taken from traditional yoga, is meant to strengthen your eyelids, which have an important role in supporting the eye.

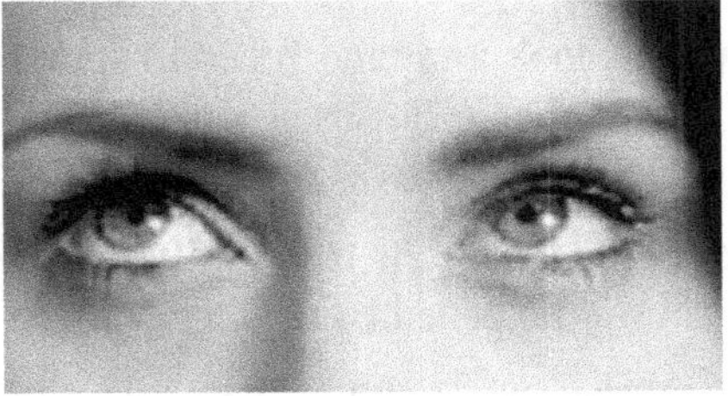

Duration: 1½ minutes

- Partially close your eyes, make sure your eyelids cover no more than half the eye.
- If your upper lids start shaking, concentrate until they stop. You can try focusing on a distant object.
- Remain in this state for 10-15 seconds, and then slowly close your eyes.
- Take a few deep breaths to increase your blood flow. Visualize that the clean air you're inhaling going into your eyes.
- Exhale, then repeat for a minute.

5. **Number 8 Movement**
This exercise will strengthen the eye muscles and will improve their flexibility.

Repetitions: 10 per direction
Sets: 3

- Imagine the number 8 lying down (∞).

- Track that shape with your eyes – do this slowly without moving your head.

- After completing 10 repetitions to one direction, blink for a few seconds, then perform 10 more repetitions to the other direction.

6. Massaging the Eyes, Temples, and eyebrows

This exercise relaxes the eyes and reduces strain and tension by increasing blood flow to these areas. Additionally, the mild pressure on the tear ducts will increase the moistness in the eyes, which provides relief for tired eyes.

Repetitions: 3

- Close your eyes.

- Lightly press on your upper eyelids and gently massage them in circular motions using 3 fingers. Perform 10 clockwise movements, and then 10 counter-clockwise movements.

- Repeat the same exercise on the lower eyelids.

- Use your fingertips to massage your temples in circular motions. Do this 20 times in a clockwise direction, and then 20 more times in a counter-clockwise direction.

- Massage the point between the eyebrows.

- Apply gentle pressure on the inner edges of the eyebrows (by the nose), and then release. Perform this exercise 3 times.

7. Controlled Cross-eyed Focusing

This exercise will strengthen your eye muscles, as well as train your eyes to focus on nearby objects, thus relieving stress on the eyes.

Duration: 5-10 Minutes

- Make a noticeable mark on a pencil.

- Hold the pencil vertically with your arm fully stretched, with the mark facing you.

- Focus on the mark, but do not proceed to step 4 until you're 100% focused on the mark.

- Slowly move the pencil closer to your face, while keeping total focus on the marked pencil. Try and maintain a straight line with your nose. Your eyes will have to adjust to keep the pencil in focus.

- Stop at the point where you start seeing double.

- Without moving your head or the pencil, look away and focus on something else, and then take a 5-second break from the exercise. If the change in focus bothers your eyes, close them for a few seconds. During this time, do not move your head or the pencil.

- Once your eyes feel rested, look back at the marked pencil, until you're fully focused on it. If it takes some time at first, don't be discouraged. If you still see the pencil twice after 2-3 tries, proceed to the next step.

- Slowly move the pencil away from your face while staying focused on it.

- Repeat for 5 minutes a day. Once this becomes easy, repeat for 10 minutes a day.

Ref: http://www.ba-bamail.com/

7 Exercises to Help Alleviate Knee Pain

If your knees are giving you problems when getting out of bed, you are not alone. Statistics show that nearly 50 million Americans feel the same way. In fact, knees are the most commonly injured joints in the body - which shouldn't come as much of a surprise, considering their everyday use, causing wear and tear. Simply walking up the stairs, for example, puts pressure on the knee joints equating to four times your body weight. But, it's never too late to alleviate knee pain. Just as a rusty door hinge can revert to its original glory with care and maintenance, your knees can be trouble free too.

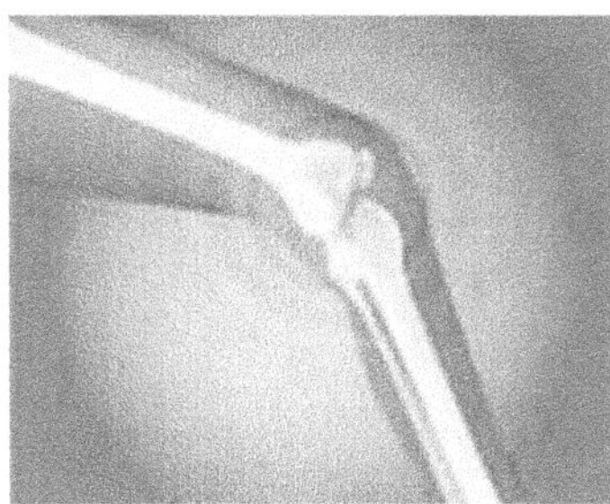

The key lies in exercising muscles surrounding the knee joints - the quadriceps (front thigh muscle), the hamstrings (back thigh muscles), the abductors (outside thigh muscles) and the adductor (inside thigh muscles).Exercising the muscles around your knee will keep them strong and less susceptible to injury. Exercising often, will also help keep your joints from stiffening, providing you with needed support, making movement easier and therefore reducing pain.

The following, simple exercises will both help you stretch and strengthen the knee area.

Straight-Leg Raise (Lying)

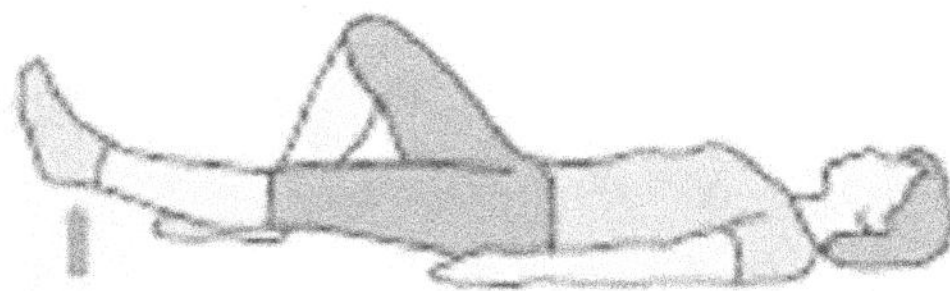

Here's How: Bend one leg at the knee, keeping the other leg straight. Lift the foot just off the floor and hold it for a slow count of 5, then lower. Repeat 5 times with each leg. For effective results, repeat this exercise in the morning and at night. You may also do so in bed.

Step Ups

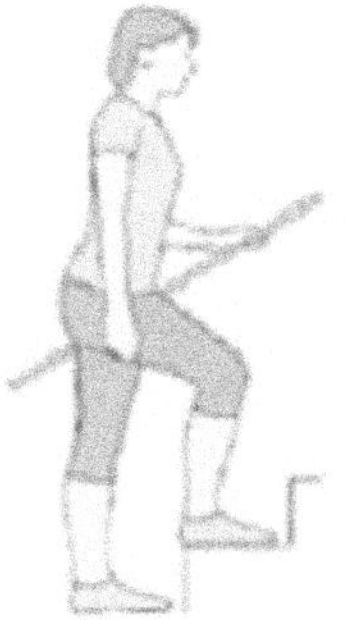

Here's How: Start at the bottom step of a staircase. Lift your left foot up on the above stair. Bring it back by your right foot. Then lower your right foot, bringing it back to neutral. Repeat, this time raising your right foot on the above stair, back to neutral, then lowering you left foot. Hold onto the banister if necessary and continue to repeat this exercise until you tire.

Knee Squats

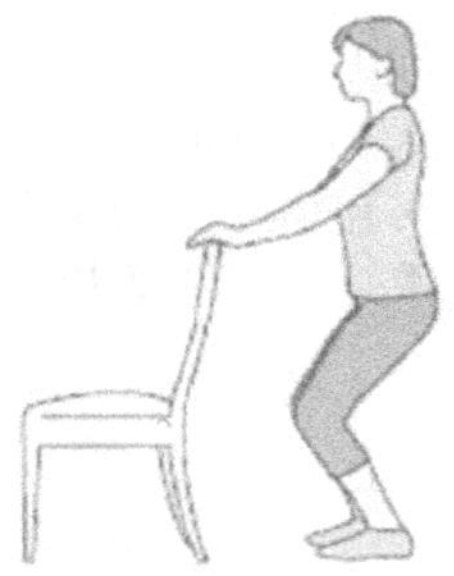

Here's How: Hold onto a chair. Squat down until your kneecap covers your big toe. Return to standing. When you are first starting, complete 10 repetitions. Then, as you improve, try to squat a little further, just be sure not to bend your knees beyond a right angle.

Leg Cross

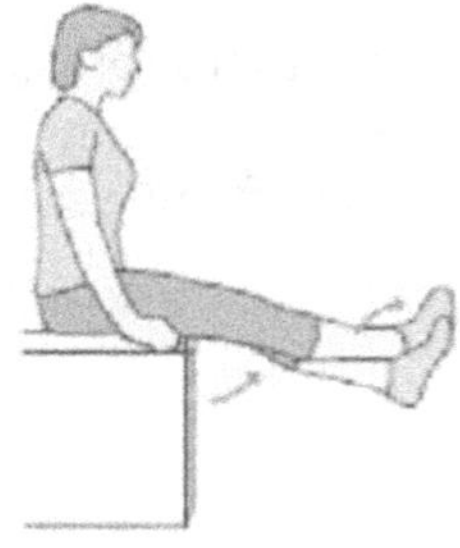

Here's How: Sit on the edge of your bed. Cross your ankles over and push your legs upwards, until your thigh muscles feel tense. Hold for 10 seconds, then relax. Switch your legs and repeat. Do 4 sets with each leg.

Leg Stretch

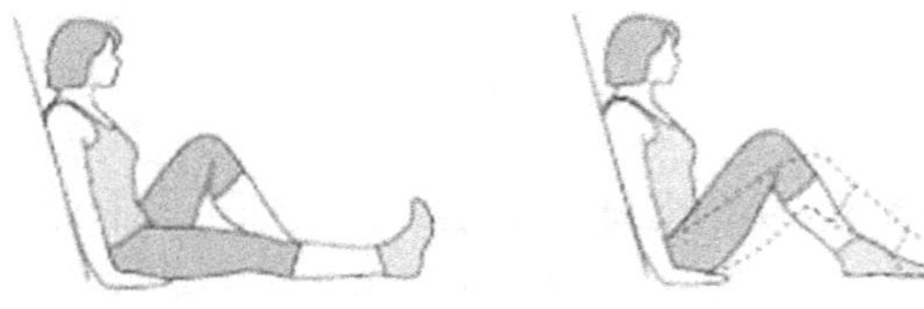

Here's How: Sit on the floor, with your legs stretched out in front of you. Slowly bend one knee, until you feel a comfortable stretch. Hold for 5 seconds. Then straighten you leg as much as you can and hold for another 5 seconds. Repeat this exercise 10 times for each leg.

Straight-Leg Raise (Sitting)

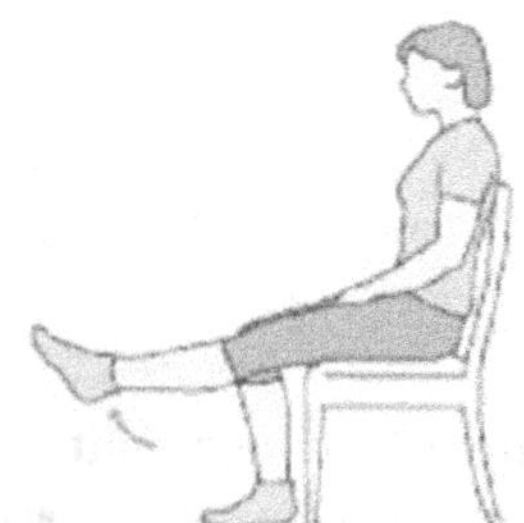

Here's How: Sit comfortably in a chair. Be aware of your posture. Straighten and raise one leg. Hold for a slow count to 10, then slowly lower your leg. Repeat 10 times with each leg. If over time, you find this easy, try the exercise with light weights on your ankles, toes pointing towards you. Do this exercise every time you sit down.

Sit/Stands

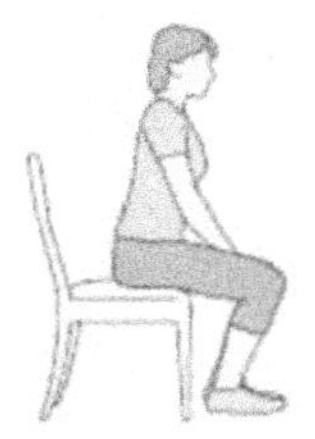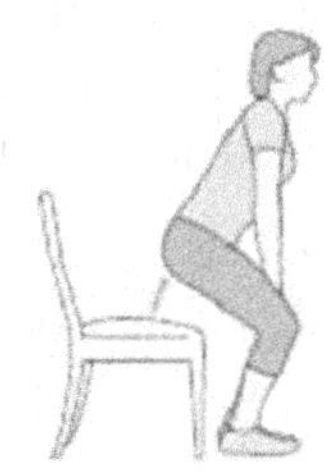

Here's How: Sit on a chair. Without using your hands for support, stand up, then sit back down. Ensure that each movement is slow and controlled. Repeat this exercise for a total of 1 minute. Over time, as you feel more comfortable, try to increase the number of sit/stands in 1 minute and try the exercise from a lower chair, or the bottom steps of a staircase.

Ref: http://www.ba-bamail.com/

7 Yoga Poses to Help with Your Sciatica Pain

Sciatica has become a common problem - if you haven't experienced it yourself, someone you know probably has. By definition, sciatica is tenderness and pain that can occur anywhere along the sciatic nerve. The sciatic nerves are the longest nerves in the human body. There are two nerves - one in each leg - originating from several nerve roots that exit from the spinal cord, passing between layers of the buttock muscles through the muscles at the back of the thigh and down through the outer edge of your leg to your foot.

The Facts: According to the Journal of Neurosurgery: Spine (2005), it is estimated that more than 5% of the adult population in the United States suffers from sciatica. Furthermore, an individual has a 40% probability of developing sciatica over a lifetime.

The Symptoms of Sciatica:
Sciatica frequently flares up when bending over, running and sitting (particularly when driving). **Symptoms for sciatica ypically include:**

- Pain in the lower back, buttocks, back of the thigh and/or calf
- Fatigue, numbness, or loss of feeling in your legs and/or feet
- Tingling, burning, pinching, pins and needles
- An inability to flex your ankles enough to walk on your heels
- Reduced reflexes in the Achilles tendon (the muscle above the heel) and the knee.

What is the Cause of Sciatica?

It is important to get to the root of the problem first and discover what is causing your sciatica. This entails seeking advice from your doctor and getting a proper diagnosis before proceeding. Generally, there are two main contributors to sciatica:
A Herniated Disk: Pain that is caused by a bulging or ruptured disk that pinches or irritates the nearby nerve.
Piriformis Syndrome: Sciatica that is caused by irritation of the sciatic nerve by a muscle in the buttocks called the piriformis. The muscle can push the sciatic nerve against the tendons beneath it, resulting in buttock and leg pain.
The Good News: How Yoga Can Help Mindful, targeted yoga practice can help you overcome the pain.
For a Herniated Disk: Opt for a yoga practice that progresses from gentle poses to basic foundational postures, which include a variation of standing poses focusing on alignment, lengthening and strengthening your lower back. Prior to practicing yoga, ensure that surgery is not required.
For Piriformis Syndrome: Opt for yoga postures that stretch this muscle. Your approach should be gentle and progressive, as overworking this muscle may lead to spasms and deep buttock pain.

What follows is a series of yoga poses that predominantly target the piriformis, helping to relieve sciatic pain:

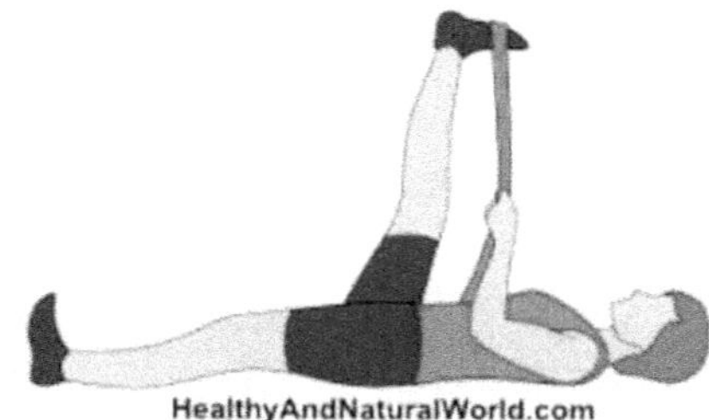

1. **Reclining Big-Toe Pose**
   Beginner's Tip: To make this pose slightly easier, raise the lower-leg heel off the floor by a few inches, or place it on a foam block or thick book for extra comfort and support. You may also use an elastic strap, placing it around the ball of your foot. Place a folded blanket under your head for added comfort.

Here's How:

- Lie on the floor, keep your legs strongly extended with your feet flexed. Exhale and bend the right knee, drawing your thigh to your torso, hugging it to your belly. Keep your left leg extended, pushing actively through the heel.

- Loop a strap around the arch of the right foot, holding the strap with both hands. On your next inhalation, extend the knee straight, pressing your heel up toward the ceiling. Reach your hands as far up the strap as possible, until your elbows are extended.

- Keep your shoulder blades broad across the back, pressing lightly into the floor. Keep your collarbones wide, reaching away from the sternum. Your sitting bones should be firmly planted on the floor.

- Hold the pose for 10 deep breaths. Then lower the leg slowly by bending the knee towards your chest and slowly releasing it to the floor. Repeat on the left side

2. Staff Pose

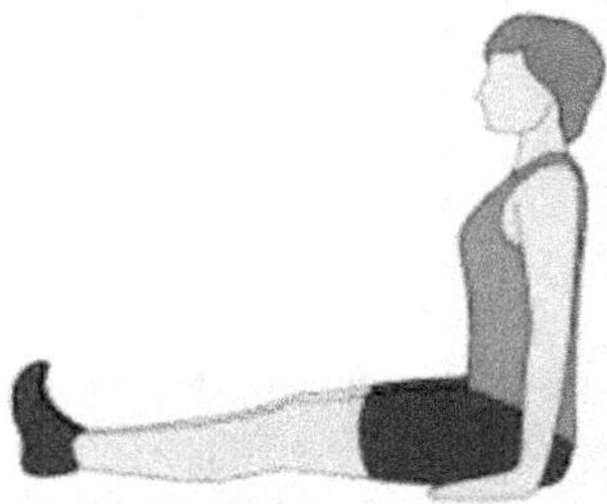

Beginner's Tip: This is a basic seated pose, which aside from relieving sciatica, will also help improve posture. Lay a 10-pound sandbag across the top of your thighs at the hip crease to help keep your thighs grounded. You may also practice this pose by keeping your back against the wall.

Here's How:

- Sit on the floor, extending both legs in front of you. Keep your legs together and your torso upright. If your torso is leaning back, sit up on a blanket or cushion to help lift your pelvis. If practicing against a wall, your sacrum and shoulder blades should touch the wall, but not the lower back or the back of the head.

- Sit on the front parts of your sitting bones, keep your thighs firm, pressing them down against the floor, rotating them slightly toward each other. Keep your ankles flexed, pressing out through your heels. Keep your spine long, as if you're being pulled by a string from the crown of your head. Hold for one minute taking long, deep breaths.

3. Pigeon Pose

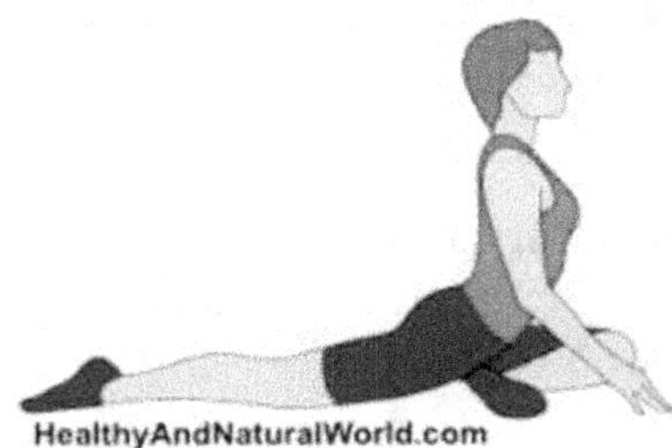

Beginner's Tip: This pose stretches the piriformis. Place a thick, folded blanket underneath you hip for extra support.
Here's How:

- Start on all fours. Bring the right knee forward and out between your hands. Slowly sink your hips to the floor. As you do so, release your left leg onto the floor behind you, slowly sliding it back while bringing your body forward. Keep your left toes pressed down on the mat.

- Your right heel should be in line with your left hip and your shin should be at about a 45 degree angle. If you feel yourself tilting over to the right hip, place a blanket underneath for extra support. Keep your hips parallel to the front of your mat as much as possible. Use your fingertips to support your torso and keep your spine long, shoulder blades drawing close together. Hold for 10 deep breaths and repeat on the other leg.

4. Standing Twist

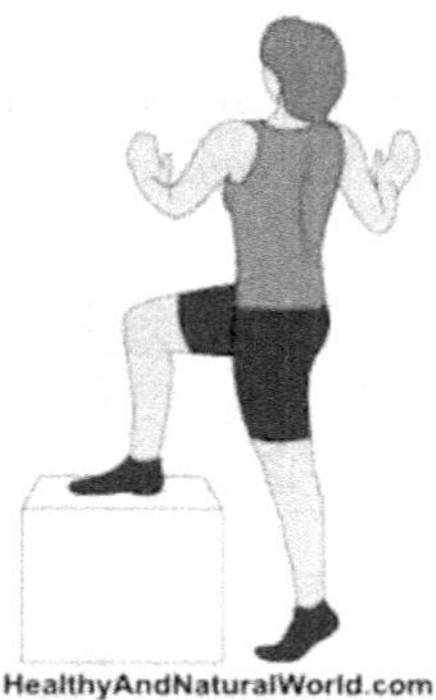

Beginner's Tip: To reap the benefits of this pose, place a chair against the wall, using both the chair and the wall for extra support, enabling you to twist deeper.

Here's How:

- Stand with your right hip against the wall with your body facing the chair. Put your right foot up on the chair, keeping your knee bent. Also keep it in line with your ankle. Your standing leg should be straight. Press your right hand against the wall, to help you balance.
- Slowly lift your left heel up and turn your torso towards the wall, supporting your hands with the wall for extra support. Exhale and lower your heel to the floor, staying in the twist for a couple more breaths. Slowly return to the starting position, repeating on your left side.

5. Preparation for Spinal Twist

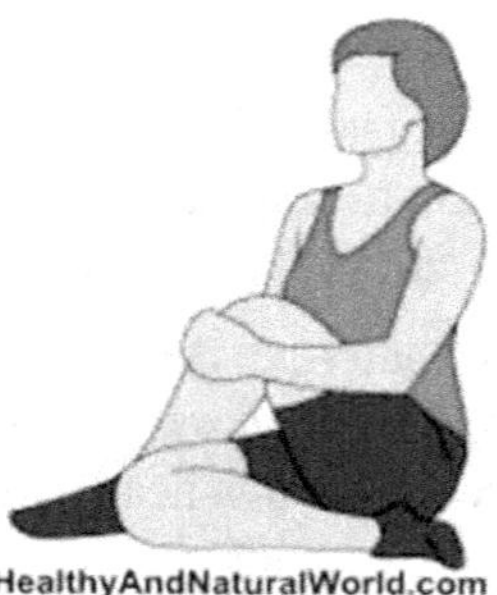

Bginner's Tip: Sit on the corner of a folded blanket for extra support in the full seated spinal twist pose (see below).

Here's How:

- Sit with your knees bent and your feet out in front of you. Release your right leg on the floor, taking your right heel to the outside of your right hip. Then bring your left foot around, placing your left heel by your right hip. Your weight should be evenly distributed across your buttocks.
- Interlock your fingers over your left knee, while focusing on lengthening your spine. Hold this position for several breaths. **Then proceed onto the next pose.**

6. Simple, Seated Twist

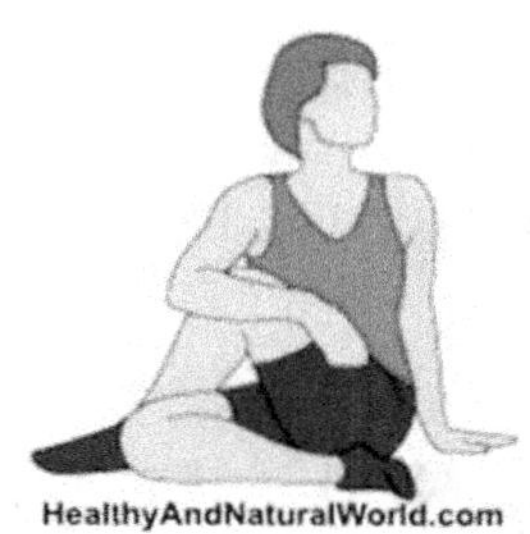

Here's How:

- From the preparation pose described above, turn your torso (from your waist, not your hip) toward the left knee. Place your left hand behind you, using it as a lever to twist (your weight should not be supported by your left arm). Hold onto your knee with your right hand.
- It is vital that you do not go too deeply into the twist, as doing so will worsen piriformis syndrome. Repeat on the opposite side, starting with the pose above.

7. Cow's Face Pose

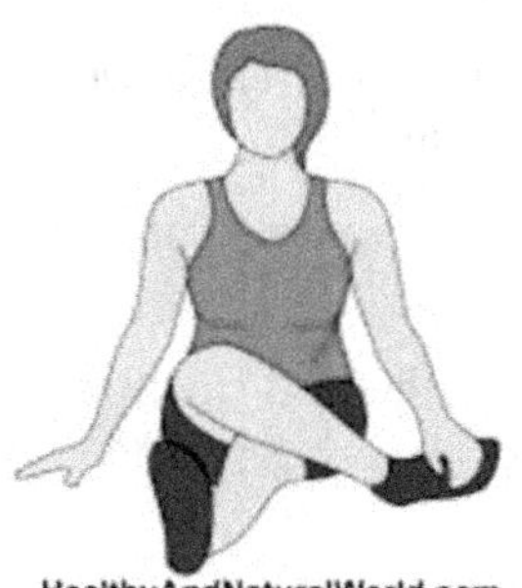

Beginner's Tip: For extra support in this passive stretch, sit on a blanket. If in the pose you notice that your left leg is not touching the floor, or the left knee locks or hurts during the stretch, roll up a second blanket or towel and place it under your knee.

Here's How:

- From staff pose (number 2), bend your right knee, bringing your right leg across the left leg. Bring your right foot close to your outer left hip.
- Move your left leg towards the mid-line - it should be slightly diagonal to your body. Your right hand should be on the floor while your left hand holds your right foot. Keep your spine extended, holding the position for a couple of breaths, then repeat on the other side.

Ref: https://yogainternational.com

7 Yoga Stretches for Your Lower Back

Do you sometimes wake up with stiff back muscles? Are certain chairs causing you pain? A sore back is a problem most people are forced to deal with at one time or another, unless they keep it strong and flexible. The following stretches come from the world of yoga, and are very effective in strengthening the lower back, as well as relieving pain in that area, the thigh muscles, knees, and shoulders.

1. The Cobra

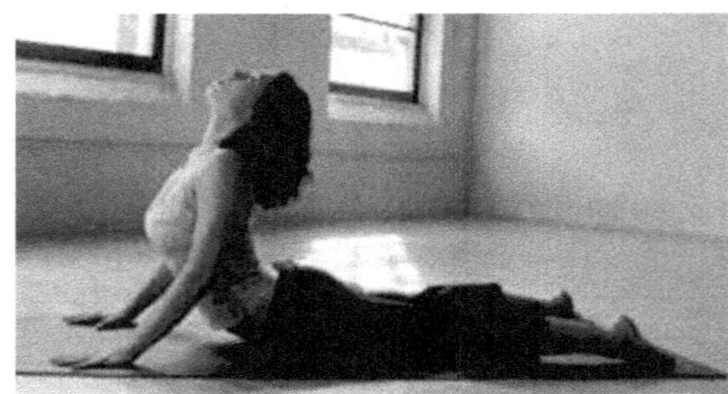

This pose improves the flexibility of the spine and stretches the chest, shoulders, and stomach.

- Lie on your stomach and put your hands forward
- Breathe in and slowly slide your hands towards your chest, while raising it and arching your back. Keep your thighs on the ground and your elbows should be slightly bent.
- Push your shoulders as far away from your ears as you can and stretch your neck. Look forward or lower your head back to maximize the stretch.
- Hold this pose for the duration of 5 long breaths, and finally exhale while you slowly lower yourself back onto the mat.

2. Child's Pose

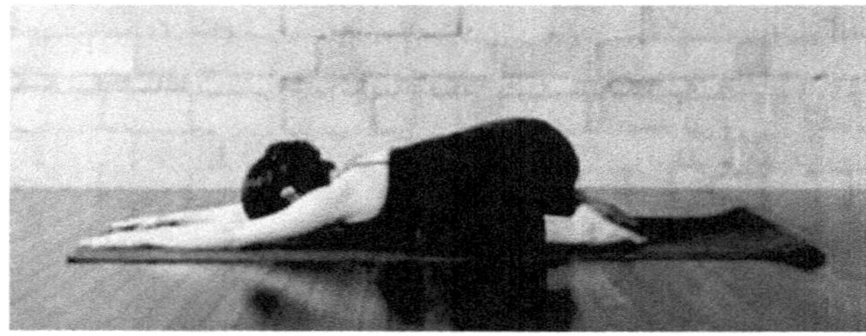

This pose complements the Cobra, and it stretches the lower back.

- Sit on your knees with your buttocks between your ankles. Support yourself with your hands. Exhale as you lower your stomach down between your knees until you're at the pose depicted in the photo above.
- Hold this pose for 5 deep, slow, breaths and exhale while returning to a sitting position.

3. Wide Squat

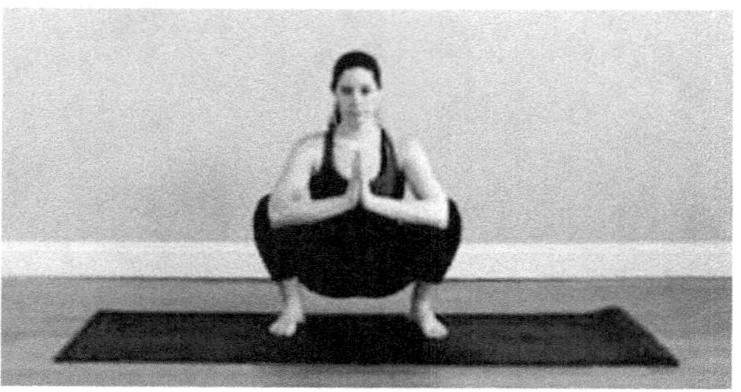

This pose helps relax the lower back, as well as ease stiff thigh muscles. It is highly recommended after a run to ease muscle tension.

- Continue from pose #2, move to a squatting position. Keep your legs spread wider than your pelvis while keeping your feet parallel.
- Push your buttocks as low as you can without touching the mat.
- Put your palms together (as shown in the photo), or put them on the floor if you need more balance. Exhale and relax your head.
- Hold this position for 5 deep, slow breaths.

4. Chest Expansion

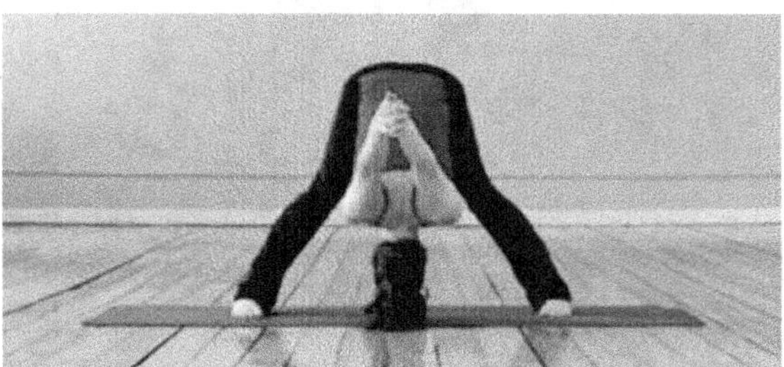

This stretch works on your chest, shoulders, lower back, and hamstrings.

- From the wide squat pose (#3), take a deep breath and move your hands behind your back. Straighten your legs, exhale slowly and bend forward.
- Slowly spread your legs wider until they're about 3 feet apart, with your heels facing out.
- Make a slight bend in your knees, until you feel the stretch in your lower back.
- Hold the pose for 5 deep, slow breaths. To improve the stretch, try pushing your hands down towards the floor.

5. Seated Straddle

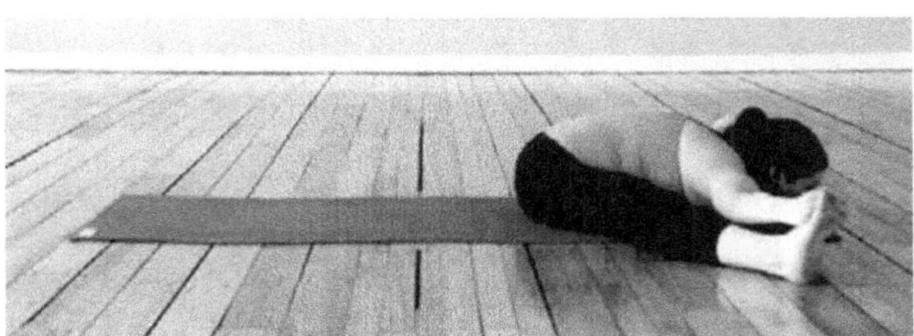

To effectively stretch your back, as well as your thighs and hamstrings, use this pose.

- Sit on the floor and spread your legs as far as they can go.
- Take a deep breath and slowly exhale while lowering your upper body towards the mat. Keep your back raight and make sure that your knees and toes are pointing up. You can place your hands on your feet or the floor.
- Stay in this position for 5 deep, slow breaths, and then slowly return to a sitting position.

6. Happy Baby Pose

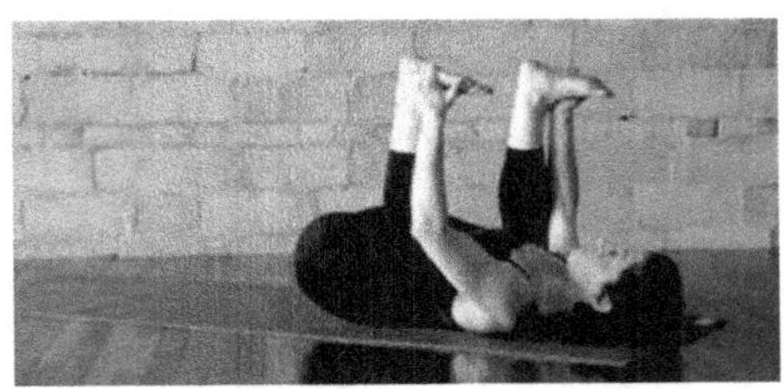

The *Happy Baby* is one of the best ways to stretch your back, and your lower back in particular. It is also useful for relaxing stiff thigh muscles.

- Lie on your back, take a deep breath, now bend your knees and pin them to your body at a 90-degree angle and hold on to your feet.
- Exhale while using your upper body to push your knees down the side of your body.
- Stay in this position for 5 deep, slow breaths and slowly release your legs.

7. Advanced: Bridge Pose

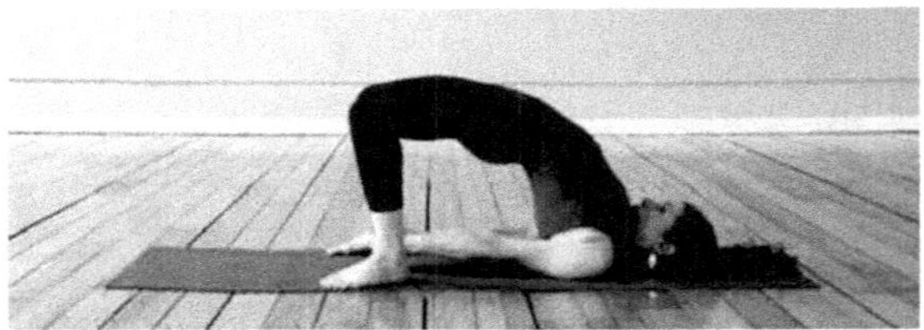

This pose will not fix your ordinary backache, but it's perfect for people with chronic back pains who want to improve the flexibility of their back and neck.

- Lie on your back and put your feet firmly on the ground. Your heels should be as close as possible to your buttocks, and at pelvic width.
- Place your hands on the floor and try to grab your ankles. If you can't, keep your arms stretched and join your fingers together. Take a deep breath and use your legs and shoulders to push up, as you raise your pelvis as high as you can.
- Keep this position for 5 deep, long breaths, and then slowly lower your pelvis down to the mat.

Ref: http://www.ba-bamail.com/

Massaging the Foot to Alleviate Headaches!

Do you want to relieve your headache in a matter of minutes? Try the ancient technique of foot massage, and feel the pain drain away. Reflexology is a simple technique performed on the feet. It is based on the belief that all major organs and nerves are connected to our feet, and by pressing in the right way on the right place, various places in our body can be cured from pain.

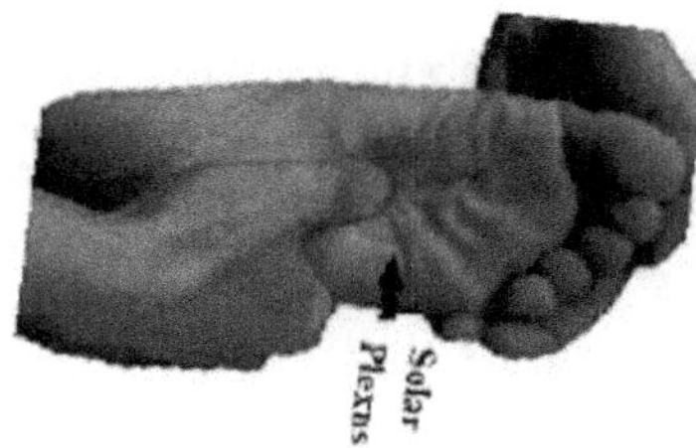

First, massaging the solar plexus is designed to relax the foot and the overall tension. This action is performed by pressing the thumb or the point of a fisted hand to the center of the foot (the solar plexus area). Gently rub for several minutes. You can also rotate the foot gently to relax the tension in the Achilles tendon.

How do you press with the thumb?

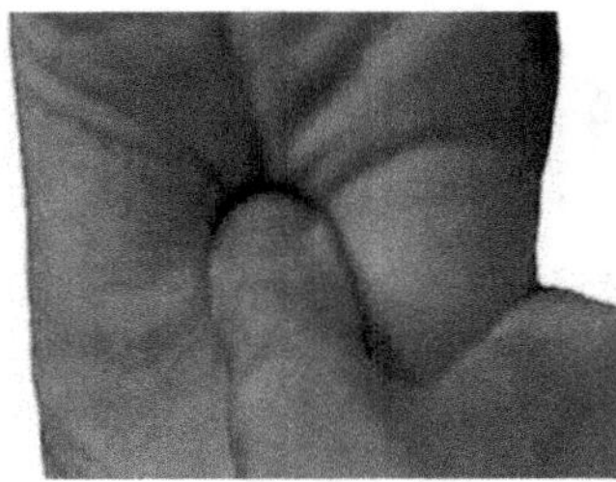

Simply press on the point and keep the thumb on it. You should use gentle pressure at first. If your thumb is a bit weak, you can use the end of a pen (not the writing tip of course) or one of the specialized reflexology tools (*see below*).

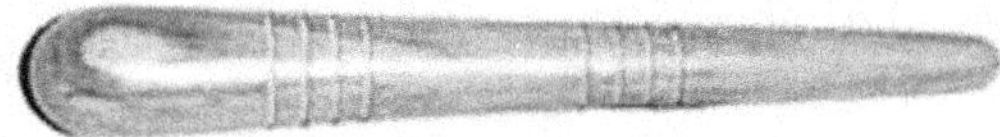

Advanced techniques require moving the thumb in a small half circle, 'walking' the thumb along different points like little steps, or just rubbing up and down, again using the thumb.

How will you be sure you found the right spot?

Usually the point of pressure will be soft, and you will feel a light sensation of being pricked. The right spot may turn a bit red, white or a little bloated, and sometimes will go numb. The right pressure is up to the point where you feel uncomfortable, but not unbearably so, and not enough to cause any damage to the skin if you are using a pen/tool.

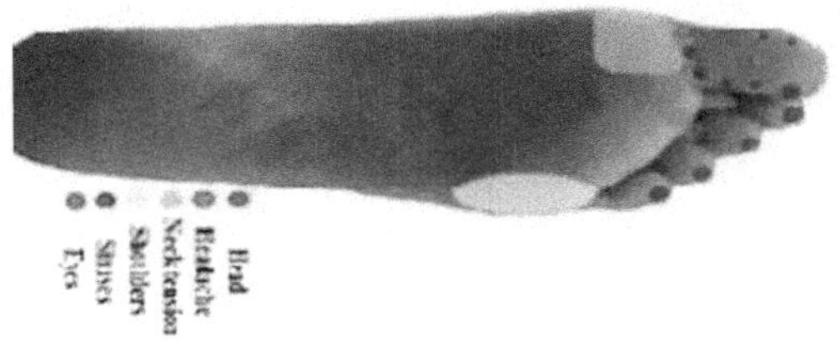

Point location

Headache caused by tension and stress - The best thing to do at first is to take a hot bath and breath deeply. Afterwards, you will need to put pressure on the inner area of the big toe, the fleshy part in the middle of it. Lastly, you'll need to put pressure on the root of the big toe..

Sinuses - The fleshy part of all the toes and the outer edges of the big toe.

Headache caused by stressing the eyes - Press and rub the root of the second and third toes.

Headache caused by tension in the neck and shoulders - Press the tip of the foot under the small toe, and the other end underneath the big toe.

Tip:

Be well hydrated to quicken the healing process and help the body get rid of accumulated toxins released by the massage. The electrolytes in the water will also help the sending of nerve conduction in the body at the same time.

Ref: http://www.ba-bamail.com/

Simple Exercises to Prevent Osteoporosis

Starting at age 30 and onwards, our bones become more porous and less dense, which makes them vulnerable to fracture, bad posture and even a shrinkage of our stature. That said, there are good ways of preventing loss of bone density through exercise. Below I will explain a bit about bone density, why we lose it with age and what exercises you can perform to maintain it.

Osteoporosis

Why does osteoporosis occur?

During our lifetime, the bones in our body are dismantled and rebuilt, but after age 30, the bone gets to a state where the deconstructed material is more prevalent than the built. This situation causes osteoporosis and damages the overall strength of our frame. The osteoporosis makes our bones vulnerable and causes possible fractures. The most common places for a fracture are in the wrist, the vertebra and the hips.

Who suffers from osteoporosis?

Because of the function estrogen plays in this process, women after menopause are the biggest sufferers of osteoporosis. That said, men also suffer from this problem. Bone density deteriorates faster in women around age 50, while with men it appears around age 70.

There are various types of medication for osteoporosis, usually given when the situation is especially bad. Still, the best known way of treating osteoporosis is prevention by exercise. Once the process of osteoporosis has already begun, exercise slowly loses effect, and so the medical recommendation is to begin regular exercise as early as possible.

8 Exercises for the prevention and treatment of osteoporosis

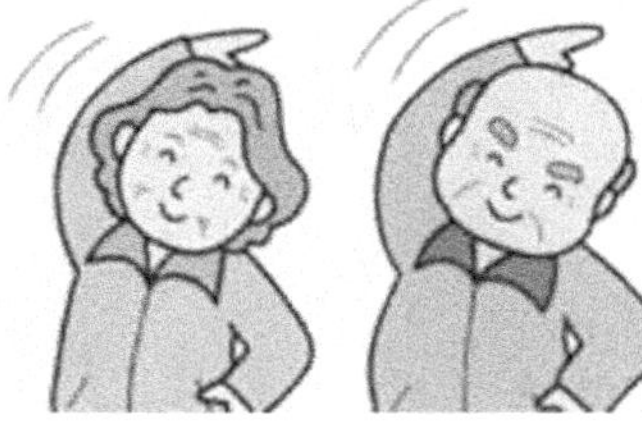

The exercises laid out here are not overly complicated, but can be performed on rising levels of difficulty. The idea is to challenge your body in order to strengthen it and remain at a rising level of difficulty. But one must understand and know what the limitations of the body are, so as to not cause damage during training. Regular, persistent exercises, rising in difficulty, will help you improve your bone density and slow down its breakage. The training should combine exercises that work on your balance, coordination, strength and flexibility.

Each exercise explained here will have a basic and advanced version. If you already suffer from osteoporosis - stick to the basic version. If you feel these exercises are too easy, slowly move to the advanced version.

During the activity, avoid stretching your spine and wrists, keep your neck and shoulders relaxed, and don't forget to breath during the exercise. After a light warm-up of walking or going up the stairs for 5-10 minutes, perform 2 sets of each exercise and rest for about 45 seconds between each set. Complete the sets of each exercise before moving on to the next. For optimal results, perform this activity 3-4 times a week, do aerobics for 30 minutes at least 3 times a week and build a diet menu rich in calcium.

Retracting Arms

<u>Works on:</u> Posture, bone strength, back and shoulder muscles.

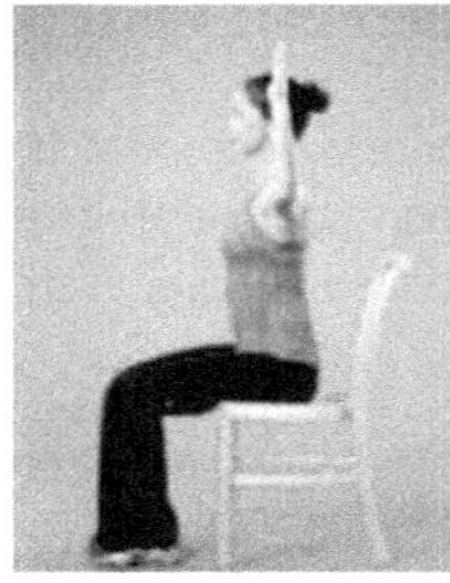 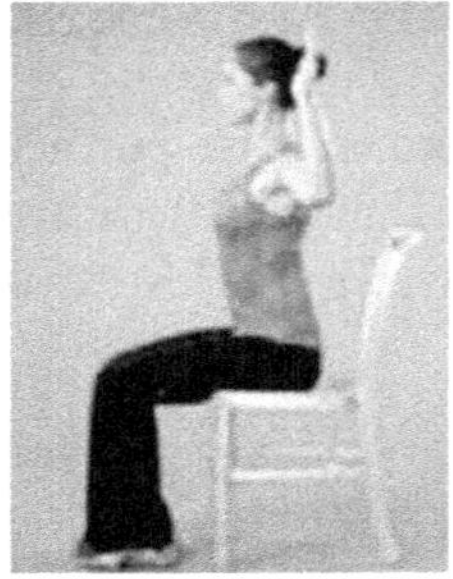

Sit with your back straight on a well-balanced, strong chair, with your feet flat on the floor.

- Lift your arms to the sides of your shoulders and hold your forearms at a 90-degree angle.
- Make sure your wrists are just above your elbows.
- Squeeze the shoulder muscles one against the other by retracting your arms back and downwards.
- Hold for 2 seconds, release and repeat.
- Don't let your head pull you forward.
- Advanced version:

Lay on your stomach and perform the same action with your arms and shoulders. Lift your arms as high as possible. Hold for 2 seconds, lower back down and repeat.

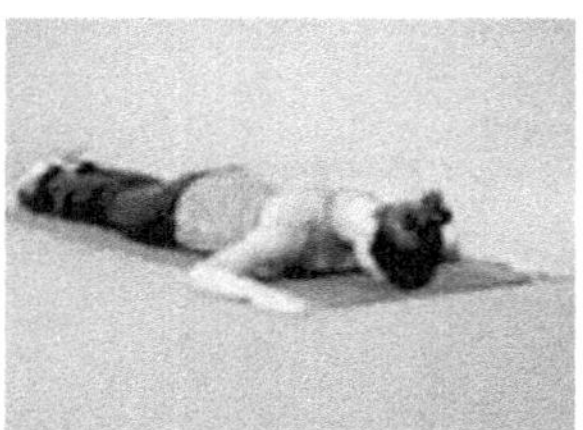 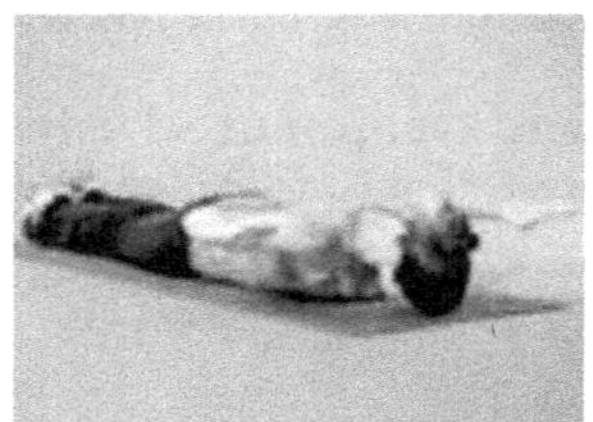

Bridge

<u>Works on:</u> Bone strength, buttocks, thigh muscles, quadriceps and hamstrings.

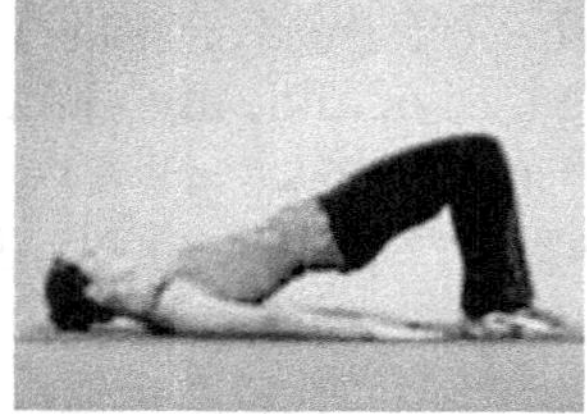 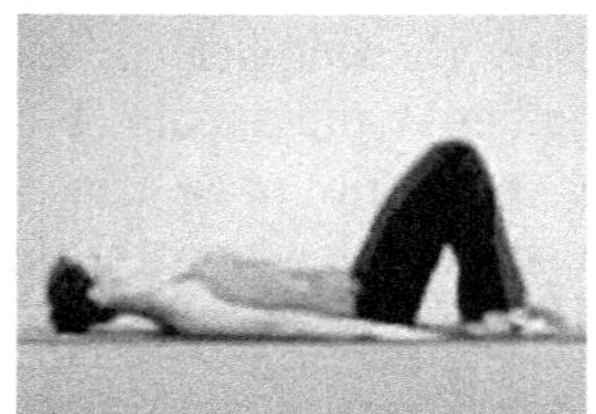

- Lay on your back with your arms at your sides and lay your feet flat on the floor with your knees bent.
- Exhale, clench your buttocks and your stomach muscles, and lift your hips as high as possible.
- Remain in this form for 1 second, return to the lying down position and repeat the action.
- Make sure that when you are raising your hips, your thighs and body form a straight line.

Advanced version:
Make things harder on yourself by crossing one leg over the knee of the other. Complete the action and change legs.

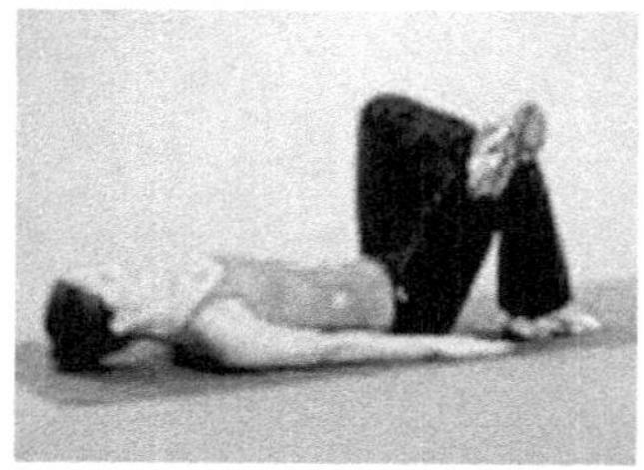 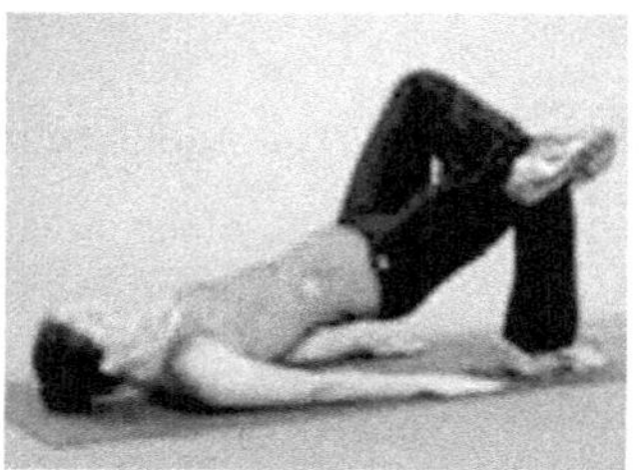

Squat

<u>Works on:</u> Balance, strengthening your hips, quadriceps and buttocks.

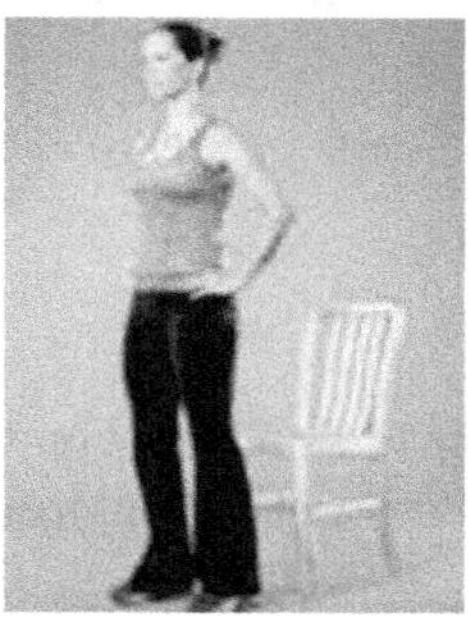 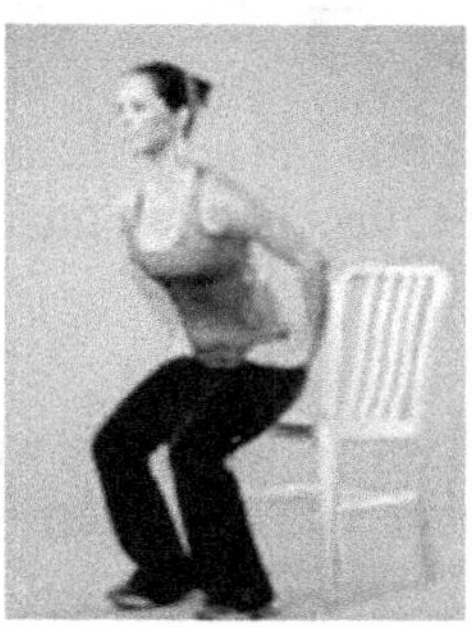

- Stand in front of a sturdy chair with your back to it.
- Slowly distance your legs from one another until they are hip wide.
- Slowly sit by bending your knees.
- Keep your knees in line with your toes.
- Stand up and repeat the movement.
- If the movement is too hard for you, put down a pillow to make the seat taller.
- Repeat 5-10 times (according to your ability) over 3 sets.

Advanced version:

Stand to the side of the chair and hold it for support. Perform a sitting movement while one leg is on the floor and the other in the air for balance. Get down to the height of the chair and slowly rise. Then change legs and repeat.

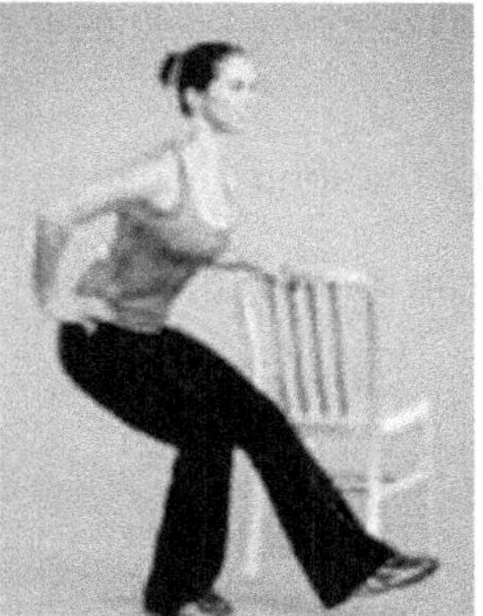

Plank

<u>Works on:</u> Balance, strengthening the wrists, bone strength and shoulder muscles.

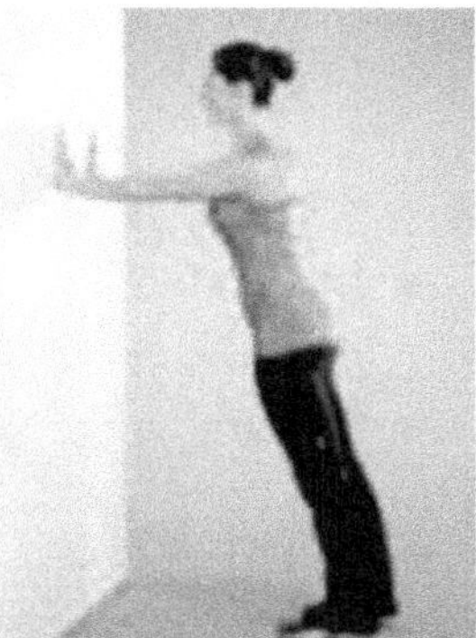

- Stand about 30 inches (80 cm) away from the wall, facing it.

- Put your hands on the wall at shoulder height and lean on the wall.

- Transfer the weight of your body to your hands.

- Keep your stomach muscles clenched and your neck aligned with your spine. Hold this position for 10 seconds, and then return to the first position.

- Try to raise the amount of time you can hold the position, until you reach 45 seconds. You can also take a little more distance from the wall to make things harder on yourself.

Advanced version:
Lie down on the floor and push yourself with your hands, with your toes anchored on the floor. The palms of your hands should be just under the shoulders. If this is too hard, start with your knees on the floor and try to work your way up to the full form.

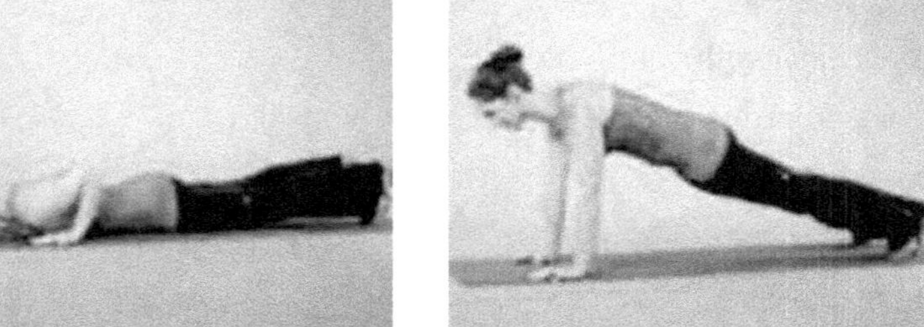

If you're interested in a more formal frame for your workout, there are other types of exercises you can integrate into your daily routine:

Tai Chi: Builds on your coordination and muscles. It is highly recommended for women. A 45 minute exercise a day, 5 times a week, can really do wonders.

Yoga: Raises the density of minerals in the spine, hip and wrist bones. It also works on your balance, coordination, concentration and bodily awareness.

Dancing: This can be an exercise that combines dancing such as zumba, but also tango or salsa dancing will do the trick and strengthen your bones.

Tennis: Mainly improves bone density in the area of the shoulders and arms, but also works on the legs and feet.

Strength training: Using free weights to exercise can contribute to bone growth. Twice a week will lead you to good results.

Ref: http://www.ba-bamail.com/

Thanks

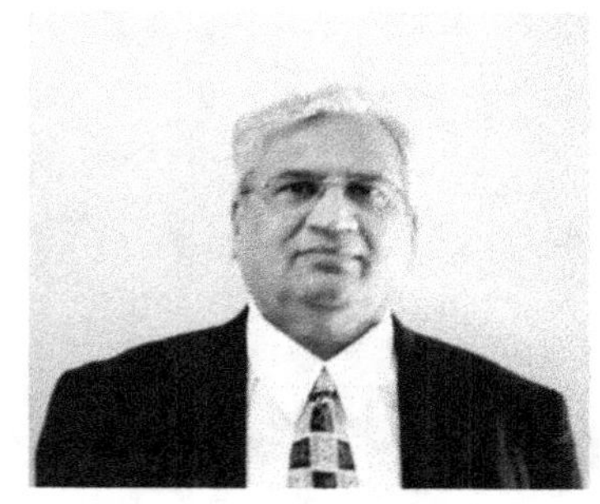

I hope you have found it interesting and useful. Do send me your suggestions and critic to make it more users friendly and useful.

Syed Shaukat Islam Rizvi

Shaukat.rizvi@gmail.com

http://ca.linkedin.com/pub/shaukat-rizvi/8/4b7/503

http://www.asc6x.org/pages/Syed-Shaukat-Islam-Rizvi.html

2021 Colonel William Parkway

Oakville   ON L6M0B8

Canada

+19052280937

+16479225925

www.ingramcontent.com/pod-product-compliance
Lightning Source LLC
Chambersburg PA
CBHW081227250726
48654CB00012B/1254